Springer Series on Child and Family Studies

The Springer Series on Child and Family Studies addresses fundamental psychological, educational, social, and related issues within the context of child and family research. Volumes published in this series examine clinical topics with an additional focus on epidemiological, developmental, and life span issues. Leading scholars explore such factors as race and immigration, parenting, and the effects of war and violence on military families and unite a vast literature into a comprehensive series of related research volumes.

More information about this series at http://www.springer.com/series/13095

Anthony A. Peguero • Jun Sung Hong

School Bullying

Youth Vulnerability, Marginalization, and Victimization

Springer

Anthony A. Peguero
Arizona State University
Tempe, AZ, USA

Jun Sung Hong
School of Social Work
Wayne State University
Detroit, MI, USA

ISSN 2570-0421 ISSN 2570-043X (electronic)
Springer Series on Child and Family Studies
ISBN 978-3-030-64366-9 ISBN 978-3-030-64367-6 (eBook)
https://doi.org/10.1007/978-3-030-64367-6

This Springer imprint is published by the registered company Springer Nature Switzerland AG
The registered company address is: Gewerbestrasse 11, 6330 Cham, Switzerland

To bullied, harassed, discriminated, victimized, and marginalized youth who endure violence, persevere in the face adversity and overcome obstacles in their pursuit to achieve success and represent their families, communities, and themselves.
To the educators, policymakers, and community stakeholders who are welcoming and committed to facilitating the well-being of ALL youth, but also with particular awareness and empathy for vulnerable and marginalized youth.
We stand with you.

Foreword

It is 2020, a quarter century after I was introduced to the pioneering scholarship on schoolyard bullying (i.e., whipping boys) of Professor Dan Olweus in Norway. As a graduate student research assistant on a federally funded youth violence prevention project at Indiana University, I remember turning to the PI Kris Bosworth encouraging her to consider developing a scale to measure school bullying. At that time, there were less than ten papers published in US-based journals on the topic of bullying in K-12 settings, and most of them were focused on students with disabilities and their experiences with bullying. We did develop a self-report measure of bullying for middle school youth, and that set us on a course to that would eventually lead to hundreds of articles, grant funding focused on the topic, and major changes to policies and practices to prevent youth bullying. It was not an easy task to convince scholars focused on youth aggression that the dynamic, the context, and very essence of bullying differed from other forms of aggression and warranted its own line of inquiry.

Indeed, I think we were successful in our efforts to encourage a concerted push a research agenda that is multidisciplinary (e.g., psychology, social work, criminology, public health, education, nursing) and specifically focused on bully prevention in our schools. Certainly, there has been a burgeoning of research focused on bullying in schools; a quick search yielded over 4000 published articles from 1995 to present. These studies have uncovered the complexity of bullying as a dynamic set of behaviors, that depends on context, that varies as a function of individual differences, familial characteristics, school-level factors, as well as neighborhood and societal level indicators. Some of these studies have systematically documented that certain populations are at elevated risk for experiencing bullying as a perpetrator, victim, or both. These include, for example, gender and sexual minority youth and students with disabilities, and research on these two populations continues to expand. However, other populations are largely ignored in the extant literature. But this book by Drs. Peguero and Hong fills this gap by highlighting how the social-ecological model can help guide the investigations of bullying among under-represented and under-studied populations and draws upon perspectives and influences beyond the individual student. For example, they open our eyes to the experiences of youth in the court systems, immigrant populations, youth and families who are struggling economically, and go further by addressing the interplay of race and ethnicity along with other marginalized identities. This inequality lens is refreshing given that much of the extant literature has not directly examined how inequities and overt racist practices in our educational systems, our juvenile court systems, our immigration policies, and fiscal policies all play out day after day on our school playgrounds, hallways, school buses, and in our homes. Thank you both for this excellent contribution to the field of bully prevention.

Dorothy L. Espelage
William C. Friday Distinguished Professor of Education
The University of North Carolina at Chapel Hill
School of Education
Chapel Hill, NC, USA

Preface

This book reviews sociological, psychological, criminological, and educational research literature pertaining to school bullying and the associated experiences in bullying and school violence among vulnerable and marginalized youth. It also examines how inequities associated with socioeconomic and social status, family cohesion and interactions, sex, sexual orientation, gender identity, and gender expression, race, ethnicity, immigration, and religion, and disabilities and special health needs are significantly associated with youth's experiences in bullying and presents how a social-ecological framework can inform the problem and address school bullying. First, this book presents a comprehensive review of school bullying research in the United States that utilized qualitative, quantitative, and mixed methods interdisciplinary and multidisciplinary research on school bullying in various interpersonal and environmental contexts. A multidisciplinary approach to understanding school bullying and victimization from the perspectives of vulnerable and marginalized youth conveys the importance of expanding our understanding of this phenomenon among various disciplines, which can bridge our gap of knowledge and enhance communications and exchange of ideas among social scientists. Our book bridges this gap in knowledge by addressing not only the individual, intrapersonal, and environmental factors but also distal-level factors and conditions that are specifically relevant to youth, such as culture and law. Second, this book is unique in that we contextualize relevant multilevel factors that foster or inhibit bullying victimization among vulnerable and historically marginalized children and adolescents who are faced with cumulative social inequality.

Tempe, AZ, USA Anthony A. Peguero
Detroit, MI, USA Jun Sung Hong

Acknowledgments

Gratitude is extended for the helpful comments and constructive suggestions from Judy Jones, Shabib Shaikh, and Nirb Singh for their steadfast encouragement, support, and patience as well as everyone at Springer and reviewers throughout the development of this book.

Anthony A. Peguero: I would like to thank Judy Jones, Shabib Shaikh, and Nirb Singh for the opportunity to publish this book and their editorship. I would like to thank my coauthor Jun Sung Hong for our collaboration with this book. We have collaborated for over a decade and it has been a great learning experience and privilege to work along with him throughout this process. A special thanks to Dorothy L. Espelage for all her research, teaching, and policy efforts with understanding and addressing bullying in the United States and globally. She has set a high standard for all of us to pursue who are seeking to ameliorate bullying and victimization in young people's lives. Appreciation is extended to Joong Won Kim, a graduate student in Sociology and graduate research associate, *Laboratory for the Study of Youth Inequality and Justice*, for his editorial assistance. On a more personal note, I would like to thank all the mentors, students, mentees, colleagues, friends, and family who have been supportive and collaborated throughout this research enterprise. I incredibly appreciate our home with a loving, supportive, adventurous, and patient partner (Dr. Jennifer M. Bondy) as well as wonderful and playful dogs (Nana, Quito, and Nola) who all remind me of the daily importance of love and laughter in life. I try my best to represent all of you with my scholarship and academic pursuits. Finally, as a child of an Ecuadorian immigrant mother and Dominican immigrant father, I acknowledge all the children of immigrants and marginalized youth who are facing, enduring, persisting against, and overcoming the challenges, hurdles, and trauma of attending unsafe school environments. Ultimately, the bullied, harassed, discriminated, victimized, and marginalized youth are the bedrock of the United States' academic and economic future.

Jun Sung Hong: I would like to express my deepest gratitude to Dr. Nirbhay Singh, Judy Jones, and Shabib Shaikh of Springer Publisher for allowing us to publish this book. I also wish to express my appreciation for Dr. Anthony A. Peguero, my lifelong colleague, for the collaboration on this book, as well as many collaborations over the years. A special thanks to Joong Won Kim, a graduate student in Sociology at Virginia Tech, for his editorial assistance. So many colleagues have been supportive in this endeavor, and it is difficult to name them all. However, I wish to thank Dr. Cheryl Waites Spellman, former Dean of the School of Social Work at Wayne State University (presently at the University of North Carolina, Charlotte), for her encouragement. I also wish to thank Dr. Jerrold (Jerry) R. Brandell, professor emeritus in the School of Social Work at Wayne State University, for his sound advice in book publications. Dr. Dorothy L. Espelage, a trailblazer in research on bias-based bullying, has been highly instrumental in advancing our understanding of how vulnerable and marginalized adolescents are affected by bullying. And finally, I wish to express my utmost appreciation to my mother (Young Hye Hong), my sister (Annie Hong), and my late father (Young Dae Hong) for a lifetime of support.

Contents

1 **Introduction to School Bullying and Inequality** 1

2 **The Relevance of the Social-Ecological Model and the Significance of Stratification** 13

3 **Status Matters: How Socioeconomic and Social Statuses Are Associated with Bullying** 23

4 **The Role of the Family: Parents/Guardians, Siblings, Cohesion, and Interactions** 39

5 **Sex, Sexual Orientation, Gender Identity, and Gender Expression: Definitions and Implications for Marginalization** 55

6 **The Color of School Bullying Victimization: Race, Ethnicity, Immigration, and Religion** 69

7 **Bullying and Youth with Disabilities and Special Health Needs: Victimizing Students with Physical, Emotional/Behavioral, and Learning Disorders** 85

8 **Bullying and Victimization of Youth in the Court Systems** 99

9 **Conclusion: Implications and Addressing School Bullying and Inequality** 113

Index 131

About the Authors

Anthony A. Peguero Dr. Anthony A. Peguero is a professor of the T. Denny Sanford School of Social and Family Dynamics and School of Criminology and Criminal Justice at Arizona State University. Dr. Peguero's research focuses on youth violence, socialization and marginalization, education, and the adaptation of the children immigrants. Overarching themes in Dr. Peguero's research include the barriers and challenges faced by the children of immigrants; how social inequality is central for sociological and criminological theories toward understanding and addressing youth violence; the intersection of race/ethnicity, immigration, and gender in relationship to youth marginalization, particularly within schools; and policies intended to promote safety and equity for youth. Dr. Peguero serves as the director of the *Laboratory for the Study of Youth Inequality and Justice*, research fellow at the *Institute for Society, Culture and Environment*, and research affiliate of the *Center for Peace Studies and Violence Prevention*. He is also a member of the *Racial Democracy, Crime, and Justice Network* and cofounder of *Latina/o/x Criminology*, which both hold the goals of advancing research on the intersection of race, crime, and justice and promoting racial democracy within the study of these issues by supporting junior scholars from under-represented groups.

Jun Sung Hong Dr. Jun Sung Hong is an associate professor in the School of Social Work at Wayne State University. He is currently the Co-Director of the Laboratory for the Study of Youth Inequality and Justice (in Virginia Tech). For the past several years, Hong has primarily conducted research on factors associated with bias-based bullying and peer victimization of racial/ethnic minority, immigrant, LGBTQ, juvenile justice-involved and economically disenfranchised adolescents and young adults in the United States and in South Korea. He has also collaborated with scholars in South Korea, Taiwan, Sweden, Scotland, Switzerland, Spain, Brazil, Ukraine, China, and Hong Kong on research projects. He is also on the scientific committee of the World Anti-Bullying Forum 2021.

Chapter 1
Introduction to School Bullying and Inequality

Abstract In this introductory Chap. 1, we provide an overview about how this book will review sociological, psychological, criminological, and educational research literature pertaining to school bullying and the associated experiences in bullying and school violence among vulnerable and marginalized youth. It also examines how inequality associated with socioeconomic and social status, family cohesion and interactions, sex, sexual orientation, gender identity, and gender expression, race, ethnicity, immigration, and religion, and disabilities and special health needs are significantly associated with youth's experiences in bullying and presents how a social-ecological framework can inform the problem and address school bullying. This book seeks to bridge gaps in knowledge by addressing not only the individual, intrapersonal, and environmental factors, but also distal level factors and conditions that are specifically relevant to youth, such as culture and law as well as contextualize relevant multi-level factors that foster or inhibit bullying victimization among vulnerable and historically marginalized children and adolescents who are faced with cumulative social inequality.

Keywords School bullying · Inequality · Patterns · Victim

Introduction

Youth violence, according to the Centers for Disease Control and Prevention, is a top public health concern, because of the long-lasting detrimental effects on the physical health and emotional well-being of youth who are victimized. Youth violence occurring within schools, in particular, has received increased attention and scrutiny over the years because schools are recognized as contexts of socialization that have direct influence on youth development, educational progress, and life-course trajectories [1–3]. In 2011, President Obama held a conference addressing the serious nature of bullying in American school districts which sparked much research interest about the causes, correlates, and consequences of school bullying. As a result of this increased research, it is evident that there are various fac-

A. A. Peguero, J. S. Hong, *School Bullying*, Springer Series on Child and Family Studies, https://doi.org/10.1007/978-3-030-64367-6_1

tors and disparities or inequalities associated with school bullying victimization which are linked to individual, family, school, community, and social and cultural characteristics and contribute to the degree of vulnerability among victimized youth. In other words, there is diversity among victims of school bullying, which reflects differences in vulnerability, marginalization, and victimization. There are diverse social factors that are reflective of privilege and power inherent in our school districts, such as socioeconomic status, family characteristics, gender, race and ethnicity, and ability status [4–7]. Thus, understanding and addressing school bullying, as an integral part of the larger problem of youth violence in schools, has become a serious concern for parents, school administrators and staff, and policymakers [1–3]. As a result of the growing number of studies exploring the correlates of school bullying, it appears that a social-ecological approach is an effective theoretical framework for understanding and addressing this phenomenon in two fundamental ways.

First, the social-ecological framework highlights the importance of considering multiple-level factors that surround individual behavior. Bullying behavior is not simply influenced by individual attitudes and behaviors but is also influenced or inhibited by interpersonal relationships, as well as broader social environmental factors such as school, community, and society at large. Ideally, schools are institutions that promote democracy and facilitate educational progress. However, historically, schools are characterized by disparities and inequalities in students' educational experiences [8, 9]. Of course, addressing the violence and bullying victimization that occurs at school for all youth is paramount; but ensuring the safety and well-being of underserved, vulnerable, and marginalized youth is particularly pressing.

Second, numerous studies have found, for example, that students' experiences in bullying and peer victimization at school are higher among racial and ethnic minority youth, sexual minority youth, and youth with disabilities than among White and heterosexual youth and youth without disabilities [see 4, 5]. Moreover, sexual minority youth who are frequently victimized are at a significantly higher risk of suicide than heterosexual youth [see 10, for a review]. Therefore, it is imperative to highlight the distinct vulnerabilities that different segments of the student population experience and endure when it comes to school bullying victimization.

In sum, this book reviews sociological, psychological, criminological, and educational research literature about school bullying and the associated experiences in bullying and school violence among vulnerable and marginalized youth. It also examines how disparities and inequalities associated with socioeconomic and social status, family cohesion and interactions, sex, sexual orientation, gender identity, and gender expression, race, ethnicity, immigration, religion, disabilities, and special health needs are significantly associated with students' experiences and presents how a social-ecological framework can inform the problem and address school bullying.

Defining School Bullying and Inequality

Before we delve into discussing how inequality matters with school bullying, it is first important to discuss our foundation, definitions, and parameters of school bullying, especially as it could pertain to vulnerable and marginalized student populations. In general, school bullying refers to victimization that occurs within schools; however, there is no consensus about what constitutes bullying and how it should be measured [1, 4, 11]. The definition of bullying as provided by Olweus [12] is often accepted as a standard term for bullying which includes the following criteria: (a) physical harm toward a person (e.g., hitting, kicking, pushing) or making fun of, excluding, and/or spreading rumors about a person, (b) victimization occurring repeatedly over time, and (c) the victims do not have equal strength or power to the bully [see also 1, 4, 11]. The complexities of identifying, defining, and measuring bullying are fundamental and have serious implications for research as well as policy. For instance, the debate and complexities associated with identifying, defining, and measuring school bullying are often associated with historical understanding, cultural acceptance aggression, and "teasing" among children and adolescents [13, 14].

Conventional school violence research often utilized a definition of student victimization guided by legal statutes of crime, such as murder, rape, assault, robbery, and theft; however, the definition of student victimization that typically applies to the adult realm is an inappropriate framework toward identifying, understanding and addressing victimization within schools [15, 16]. Given different psychological and sociological circumstances, the effects of victimization and harm from the violence that youth endure are comparatively more damaging to children's development than to adults [16, 17]. Research indicates that youth have limited mental capacity and are less able to defend and protect themselves than adults [16, 18]. A less severe instance of harm or victimization may cause a child to suffer emotional, mental, and physical injury where an adult would not [16, 19]. With this perspective, developmental researchers drew into question the school's culture of tolerance for behaviors, such as bullying, sexual harassment, racial/ethnic bias treatment, body image, religious persecution, and the like among the student body but also from administrators, faculty, and staff [4, 20]. Such behaviors, as well as the social and cultural practices or policies that sustain these behaviors, are consequently no longer tolerated as a normal part of the school experience for students but rather tend to be more strongly scrutinized than in the past [1, 14].

This definitional issue of school bullying is one that confronts researchers and policymakers because, in practicality, multiple definitions and associated measures permeate the literature. From a research perspective, this lack of a common standard has produced confusion concerning the prevalence of bullying as well as disagreement about what constitutes bullying. Not having a standard definition and commonly agreed threshold of school bullying across contexts may have resulted in school administrators, faculty, and staff relying on social and cultural biases to guide their interpretations and responses to bullying [6, 14, 21].

Undoubtedly, there is a wide array of potential individual and contextual factors that influence not only how school administrators, faculty, and staff define school bullying and a threshold for aggression but students as well. For instance, individual factors such as age (e.g., elementary, middle, or high school) and victim-offender relationship (e.g., siblings or dating) as well as school-level factors such as locale (e.g., urban or suburban) and size of the school are just some of the many known factors that influence how school administrators, faculty, staff, and students define, understand, report, and respond to school bullying.

We should mention, however, that the relationship between bullying and victimization is symbiotic, especially within school contexts. For example, Melde and Esbensen [22] examined a nationally representative sample of 250 schools and found that engagement in school-based misbehavior is a strong predictor of school-based victimization. In other words, victimization and offending, albeit two distinct phenomena, will be at times conflated because both are known to have derailing influence on positive development and educational progress [5, 16, 23]. Although we acknowledge this close relationship, the focus of this book will be on bullying victimization. As noted, the power imbalance is fundamental in the definition of bullying. As a consequence, inequalities in defining who is considered a victim of school bullying have emerged as well as recognizing that marginalized and vulnerable segments of the student population have increased odds of being victims of bullying and violence at school.

Of course, addressing violence and bullying that occurs within schools for all students is paramount toward sustaining a system that is supposed to facilitate educational progress and sustainability; however, acknowledging and addressing the inequalities associated with bullying appears to be a pressing step toward attaining educational justice. There is a persistent history of social and educational stratification or inequality linked to socioeconomic status, family characteristics, gender, race and ethnicity, and ability status in schools. It is thus logical that school bullying is stratified by race and ethnicity, immigration, gender, and sexual orientation, as well as other detrimental economic, social, and educational characteristics. The social problem of bullying within schools is complex as well as diverse. The research presented in this book will suggest that if policymakers, school administrators, and community stakeholders are seeking to address and ameliorate bullying within schools, it is vital to consider the significance of inequality.

Intersectionality and Implications

Intersectionality is a conceptual approach to studying the relationships across multiple dimensions and modalities of social relationships and identities such as gender, socioeconomic status, race, and ethnicity [6, 14, 24]. For example, the concept of the intersectionality of socioeconomic status, gender, race, ethnicity, or sexual orientation is particularly pertinent to the growing body of research on school bullying victimization [6, 14, 24]. Several researchers have argued that violence is fundamentally associated with socioeconomic status, gender, race, ethnicity, or sexual orientation which indicates that intersectionality warrants further critical analysis [6, 14, 24]. Thus, because previous research studies indicate that intersectionality with social inequalities is important toward understanding the occurrence of school bullying victimization, we encourage you to not simply read each chapter and topic as mutually exclusive, but rather be critical by utilizing how these distinct inequalities intersect with each other when understanding bullying victimization throughout this book.

The Growing Significance of Social Inequality in School Bullying

Problems and responses to school bullying are popular topics among the news media, schools, politicians, communities, families, and other stakeholders. News reports and articles describing narrowly avoided school bullying tragedies, as well as those about incidents that occur and their tragic consequences (e.g., suicide), appear almost daily. Yet, there have been surprisingly few efforts to understand how our efforts to address and ameliorate school bullying do not consider the diversity of students and inequities for vulnerable and marginalized youth. As a result, many of the programs and policies implemented across school districts have been characterized as "one size fits all", with little evidence of effectiveness [5, 6, 25]. Thus, we hope that this book can present evidence-based findings that can inform a wide array of individuals, including scholars, educators, policymakers, practitioners, parents, and stakeholders who are committed to addressing youth violence occurring within schools.

In this book, we present a comprehensive review of school bullying research in the United States that utilizes qualitative, quantitative, and mixed methods interdisciplinary and multi-disciplinary research on school bullying in various interpersonal and environment contexts (i.e., family relationships, peer relations, school climate, neighborhood environment, cultural forces). A multi-disciplinary approach to understanding school bullying and victimization from the perspectives of vulnerable and marginalized youth conveys the importance of expanding our understanding of this phenomenon among various disciplines, which can bridge our gap of knowledge and enhance communications and exchange of ideas among social scientists. Furthermore, although researchers over the years have made significant advances in enhancing our understanding of school bullying and victimization among racial and ethnic minorities, immigrants, Lesbian, Gay, Bisexual, Transgender, Queer or Questioning (LGBTQ), and other marginalized or vulnerable youth, much of the research has focused primarily on an individual level (e.g., attitudes, behaviors) and immediate environment factors (e.g., school climate). As a result, much of the intervention and prevention efforts have targeted individual behavior and the immediate environment (e.g., change in school climate).

Our book bridges this gap in knowledge by addressing not only the individual, intrapersonal, and environmental factors but also distal level factors and conditions that are specifically relevant to youth, such as culture and law. Although many theoretical approaches have been employed to understand and address school bullying, a socio-ecological approach is the most comprehensive; one that allows for an examination of the confluence of multiple-level factors that directly and indirectly affect youth and their vulnerability to being bullied. While the issue of school bullying has been studied to understand causes, correlates, effects, and interventions, few, if any, studies have explored the significance of social stratification. We contextualize relevant multi-level factors that foster or inhibit bullying victimization among vulnerable and historically marginalized and vulnerable students who are faced with cumulative risk, barriers, and hurdles within the school. For instance, certain factors, such as lack of diverse school climate, may reinforce social disparities, which in turn may be associated with an increased likelihood of bullying and peer victimization among the youth of color. Likewise, broader level factors, such as the current conservative political environment, may increase the unequal treatment of LGBTQ youth, which in turn may increase their risk of being bullied by peers. A comprehensive overview of diverse forms of social disparities that are pervasive in American school districts can result in more effective violence prevention strategies for vulnerable and marginalized youth. Throughout each chapter, we will examine how disparities and inequalities matter in the social-ecological approach toward understanding and addressing the issue.

Organization and Argument of the Book

In Chap. 2 titled "The Relevance of the Social-Ecological Model and the Significance of Inequality," we establish the parameters of the theoretical framework. We detail how diversity in disparities matters when utilizing the social-ecological framework. Bronfenbrenner [26–28] hypothesized that to understand youth development, one must consider the multiple social environments in which development occurs. Under this theoretical framework, Bronfenbrenner [26–28] argues that youth's development occurs within a context of the system of relationships that form their social environments. In this paradigm the social environment can be distinguished by five subsystems (i.e., societal, community, institutional, group, and individual) and that each subsystem depends on the contextual nature of a youth's life. García Coll and colleagues [29] argue, however, that researchers must consider the significance of social stratification and inequality when investigating the connections between social environment and youth development. García Coll and colleagues [29] denote that extending Bronfenbrenner's [26] social-ecological theoretical approach should consider: (1) social position (e.g., race, class, and gender), (2) social stratification (e.g., biased treatment), (3) promoting or inhibiting environments (e.g., school), (4) adaptive culture and current demands (e.g., assimilation or acculturation), (5) youth characteristics (e.g., age, psychological characteristics), and (6) family (e.g., structure, functioning) when investigating the role that the social environment has for marginalized youth. In the final section of this chapter, we introduce the key concepts to follow in subsequent chapters.

In Chap. 3 titled "Status Matters: How Socioeconomic and Social Statuses Are Associated with Bullying," we discuss how socioeconomic and social statuses are associated with bullying victimization. Low socioeconomic status, particularly living in poverty, is a risk factor for violence exposure in low-income communities and the schools that are embedded within them. In general, impoverished youth are significantly more likely to be exposed to peer violence and bullying victimization in school and are also likely to identify with a culture of violence. Low-income youth are also more likely to hold positive attitudes toward peer aggression and bullying. Since Coleman's The Adolescent Society [30], researchers have consistently found that social groups or statuses in school are important about experiences, expectations, and interactions. Social statuses such as "preppies/rich kids," "geeks/nerds," "jocks/athletes," remain as meaningful in schools today as they were five decades ago when Coleman first reported their significance. In turn, there is a long history of peer aggression, conflict, and bullying that occurs among social groups and statuses. In other words, a youth's social status in school can be linked to his or her likelihood of being bullied. Students with low social acceptance, high social rejection, or those who are labeled as nonaggressive are more likely to be victimized in school. Additionally, "smart" youth or "geeks or nerds" are perceived as weak and usually get picked on more often; whereas athletes, who are perceived as more capable of protecting themselves, are not. Research suggests that a student's popularity and friendships or social networks can be linked to the likelihood of bullying victimization and aggression that student experiences at school. It is argued that "popular" kids and/or students are usually insulated from peer victimization because they have more friends. Moreover, they are also likely to bully or encourage their peers to target an individual for bullying. We will also present how socioeconomic and social statuses need to be considered in the phenomenon of bullying victimization through a social-ecological framework.

In Chap. 4 titled "The Role of the Family: Parents/Guardians, Siblings, Cohesion, and Interactions," we demonstrate how the role of the family, specifically parents/guardians, siblings, cohesion, and interactions affect the likelihood of being bullied. Several aspects of the home environment may be particularly relevant for victims of school bullying, as they may promote resilience in children going through this stressful experience. Studies have found that family social support is an important protective factor that can mitigate the effects of bullying victimization. Youth in caring, sensitive, and safe families and home environments are less likely to experience bullying victimization in school. Youth who are rejected or bullied by their peers, but who have warm and caring parents/guardians showed fewer behavioral problems than other affected youth. Bullied youth who have strong and intimate bonds or relationships with their parents/guardians might have more favorable psychosocial outcomes than would otherwise be the case. As for siblings, strong and healthy relationships with brothers and sisters may help to buffer youth from being bullied by providing an additional source of social support. On the other hand, family factors, such as negative adult and sibling influences, lack of parental involvement, bullying among siblings, and lack of parental support, maltreatment, and unhealthy family interactions are associated with bullying victimization. It is argued that youth from families with a culture of violence or maltreatment may feel powerless, as they are unable to protect themselves from harm and bullies. These youth are also likely to develop poor social skills, making them targets of bullying victimization and social exclusion. In the final section of this chapter, we will present how the role of the family with bullying should be considered through a social-ecological framework.

In Chap. 5 titled "Sex, Sexual Orientation, Gender Identity, and Gender Expression: Definitions and Implications for Marginalization," we examine how sex, sexual orientation, gender identity, and gender expression are linked to the likelihood of being bullied. Of course, it will be important to define the terms sex, sexual orientation, gender identity, and gender expression for our readers. Biological sex, as defined by female or male, is often the focus of bullying research and disparities are often reported with distinct forms of bullying. For instance, some research evidence suggests that girls are more likely to be victims of verbal aggression, insults, gossip, manipulation, and social isolation by their peers, while boys are more likely to be victims of physical aggression. In terms of sexual orientation, lesbian, gay, and bisexual, transgender, and sexually questioning (LGBTQ) youth are more likely to be bullied in schools than are heterosexual youth. Nearly half of LGBTQ youth report experiencing physical harassment at least once because of their sexual orientation and just over half report feeling unsafe at their school for the same reason. In terms of gender identity, boys, in general, are commonly victims and perpetrators of direct physical forms of school bullying, while girls experience indirect bullying (e.g., social rejection, relational aggression). However, findings on sex differences in bullying involvement have been inconsistent, and more recent studies report that gender was not a significant predictor. Interestingly, recent studies also found that relational aggression is not exclusively a female form, and there is little difference between the sexes in relational aggression. Moreover, transgender and transsexual youth experience difficulties that are not directly associated with their transgender status, but stem from stigma, rejection, and victimization by parents, peers, school staff, and others. Limited studies have also indicated that transgender youth face even more marginalization than their LGB peers, and have less access to remedies because many policies designed to protect LGB individuals do not provide protections for transgender youth. In terms of gender expression, researchers argue that the localized construction of masculinity/femininity plays a major role in the reflexive decision to engage in or avoid reactive violence and bullying amongst peers. It is suggested that sexual or physical violence and bullying amongst youth reflects a strategy to validate or invalidate their subordinate masculine/feminine status (internalized in the school setting) and (re)construct a dominant masculine/feminine self. In the final section of this chapter, we will present how sex, sexual orientation, gender identity, and gender expression with school bullying should be considered through a social-ecological framework.

In Chap. 6 titled "The Color of School Bullying Victimization: Race, Ethnicity, Immigration, and Religion," we explain how race, ethnicity, immigration, and religion are associated with school bullying. Most school bullying research has focused on the differential patterns of victimization between White American and African American youth. Research reveals that African American, Latino American, Asian American, and White American youth experience school bullying victimization distinctly differently. Several potential reasons have been suggested for why racial and ethnic minority youth have increased exposure to school bullying. These students are more likely to attend urban schools with higher levels of disorder and violence. Racial and ethnic minority youth are also more likely to report the presence of gangs in their schools and are more likely to report being fearful of an attack at or on the way to or from school. Some researchers suggest that inconsistencies in the patterns of racial and ethnic minority youth are associated with immigration status. Immigrant youth are often subjected to negative treatment such as discrimination, ridicule, and harassment from other students, teachers, and school administrators. Moreover, perceptions of low academic ability, rejection by peers, and fear of safety are all reflective of immigrant youth experiences within the United States school system. Additionally, the events of September 11, 2001, resulted in a dramatic increase in the bullying victimization, harassment, verbal and physical threats toward youth who are or are perceived to be Muslim in school. In the final section of this chapter, we will present how race, ethnicity, immigration, and religion with school bullying should be considered through a social-ecological framework.

In Chap. 7 titled "Bullying and Youth with Disabilities and Special Health Needs: Victimizing Students with Physical, Emotional, and Learning Disorders," we discuss how and why youth with disabilities and special health needs are vulnerable to bullying at school. Research suggests that youth with learning and developmental disabilities are at an elevated risk of peer victimization. Youth with observable disabilities in segregated settings are more likely to be victimized by their peers without disabilities in school than those with non-observable disabilities. Additionally, youth with disabilities experience victimization in school because they may be too passive or exhibit responses that may reinforce bullying behavior. Youth with learning disorders have difficulty interpreting verbal and non-verbal communication and may have poor social skills as well, which can hamper their ability to effectively establish peer relations. However, bullying incidents involving youth with disabilities are difficult to identify because these youth are less likely to have learned about abuse awareness and potential responses, which makes detection and reporting of bullying among this population a serious concern. Psychosocial problems, such as depression and anxiety, are also factors related to the likelihood of being bullied at school. Depressed youth are more likely to be victimized by their peers than are children without a history of depression. In the final section of this chapter, we will present how disability and special health needs with school bullying should be considered through a social-ecological framework.

In Chap. 8 titled "Bullying and Victimization of Youth in the Court System", we discuss how and why youth who are involved in the juvenile justice system and child welfare system are prone to bullying and peer victimization. Research suggests that youth who are detained in juvenile correctional facilities are seriously at risk of bullying and peer victimization as these youth have opportunities to affiliate with peers who engage in such behavior. Also, a large body of research literature has demonstrated a positive association between delinquent behavior and bullying and victimization, which is also supported by several theoretical perspectives, including the routine activities theory, social learning theory, and attachment theory. Although research on bullying involvement of adolescents in the child welfare system is rare, youth who are placed in out-of-home care (e.g., foster care, kinship care, group home, or residential treatment facility) are also prone to bullying and victimization, as they are typically removed from their home due to allegations of maltreatment; as a result, these youths are likely to have difficulty in socialization and forming bonds with "conventional" peers and are likely to be victimized or socially excluded.

In the concluding Chap. 9 titled "Conclusion: Implications and Addressing School Bullying and Inequality," we discuss why ameliorating violence and victimization should be a priority. Of course, addressing bullying victimization that occurs within schools for all youth is paramount toward sustaining a system that is supposed to facilitate educational progress and sustainability. However, acknowledging and addressing social stratification associated with bullying victimization appears to be a pressing step toward attaining social and educational justice. There is a persistent history of disparities linked to socioeconomic and social status, family cohesion and interactions, sexual orientation, gender identity, and gender expression, race, ethnicity, immigration, and religion, and disabilities and special health needs in the U.S. school system. The social problem of bullying within U.S. schools is both complex and diverse. It is clear that the sources and factors associated with the vulnerability and marginalization of youth to being victimized at school presented in this book also intersect. Although homes, schools, and neighborhoods may never be completely bully-free environments, there are several ways to assist students in breaking the bullying and peer victimization cycles. The first step is to take the social-ecological framework seriously and begin to create new programs or to modify existing bullying prevention programs that target more than individual characteristics and consider the complex interrelations between the individual and the various system levels. In doing so, we can help develop a healthy school environment. In addition to the social-ecological approach, it is fundamental to consider disparities and inequality that are associated with violence and victimization occurring within schools when implementing such programs. The information presented in this book is also one calling for advocacy, which will suggest that if policymakers, school administrators, and community stakeholders are seeking to address and ameliorate bullying within schools, it is vital to consider the significance of various forms of social inequality.

References

1. Bradshaw, C. P. (2017). *Handbook on bullying prevention: A life course perspective.* NASW Press.
2. Espelage, D. L., & Swearer, S. M. (2003). Research on school bullying and victimization: What have we learned and where do we go from here? *School Psychology Review, 32*(3), 365–383.
3. Hymel, S., & Swearer, S. M. (2015). Four decades of research on school bullying: An introduction. *American Psychologist, 70*(4), 293.
4. Hong, J. S., & Espelage, D. L. (2012). A review of research on bullying and peer victimization in school: An ecological system analysis. *Aggression and Violent Behavior, 17*(4), 311–322.
5. Hong, J. S., Peguero, A. A., Choi, S., Lanesskog, D., Espelage, D. L., & Lee, N. Y. (2014). Social ecology of bullying and peer victimization of Latino and Asian youth in the United States: A review of the literature. *Journal of School Violence, 13*(3), 315–338.
6. Peguero, A. A. (2012). Schools, bullying, and inequality: Intersecting factors and complexities with the stratification of youth victimization at school. *Sociology Compass, 6*(5), 402–412.
7. Watts, I. E., & Erevelles, N. (2004). These deadly times: Reconceptualizing school violence by using critical race theory and disability studies. *American Educational Research Journal, 41*(2), 271–299.
8. Gamoran, A. (2001). American schooling and educational inequality: A forecast for the 21st century. *Sociology of Education, 74*, 135–153.
9. Kozol, J. (2012). *Savage inequalities: Children in America's schools.* Broadway Books.
10. Hong, J. S., Espelage, D. L., & Kral, M. J. (2011). Understanding suicide among sexual minority youth in America: An ecological systems analysis. *Journal of Adolescence, 34*(5), 885–894.
11. Espelage, D. L., & Swearer, S. M. (2010). *Bullying in North American schools.* Routledge.
12. Olweus, D. (1993). *Bullying at school: What we know and what we can do.* Oxford, UK: Blackwell Publishers.
13. Keltner, D., Capps, L., Kring, A. M., Young, R. C., & Heerey, E. A. (2001). Just teasing: A conceptual analysis and empirical review. *Psychological Bulletin, 127*(2), 229.
14. Pascoe, C. J. (2011). *Dude, you're a fag: Masculinity and sexuality in high school.* University of California Press.
15. Gottfredson, D. C. (2001). *Schools and delinquency.* New York: Cambridge University Press.
16. Finkelhor, D. (2014). *Childhood victimization: Violence, crime, and abuse in the lives of young people.* New York: Oxford University Press.
17. McDougall, P., & Vaillancourt, T. (2015). Long-term adult outcomes of peer victimization in childhood and adolescence: Pathways to adjustment and maladjustment. *American Psychologist, 70*(4), 300.
18. Macmillan, R. (2001). Violence and the life course: The consequences of victimization for personal and social development. *Annual Review of Sociology, 27*(1), 1–22.
19. Macmillan, R., & Hagan, J. (2004). Violence in the transition to adulthood: Adolescent victimization, education, and socioeconomic attainment in later life. *Journal of Research on Adolescence, 14*(2), 127–158.
20. Thapa, A., Cohen, J., Guffey, S., & Higgins-D'Alessandro, A. (2013). A review of school climate research. *Review of Educational Research, 83*(3), 357–385.
21. Hong, J. S. (2009). Feasibility of the Olweus bullying prevention program in low-income schools. *Journal of School Violence, 8*(1), 81–97.
22. Melde, C., & Esbensen, F.-A. (2009). The victim-offender overlap and fear of in-school victimization: A longitudinal examination of risk assessment models. *Crime & Delinquency, 55*(4), 499–525.
23. Nofziger, S. (2009). Deviant lifestyles and violent victimization at school. *Journal of Interpersonal Violence, 24*(9), 1494–1517.
24. Espelage, D. L. (2016). Sexual orientation and gender identity in schools: A call for more research in school psychology—No more excuses. *Journal of School Psychology, 54*, 5–8.

25. Wilcox, P., Tillyer, M. S., & Fisher, B. S. (2009). Gendered opportunity? School-based adolescent victimization. *Journal of Research in Crime and Delinquency, 46*(2), 245–269.
26. Bronfenbrenner, U. (1979). *The ecology of human development: Experiments by nature and design*. Cambridge, MA: Harvard University Press.
27. Bronfenbrenner, U. (1986). Ecology of the family as a context for human development: Research perspectives. *Developmental Psychology, 22*(6), 723.
28. Bronfenbrenner, U. (1994). Ecological models of human development. In T. Husen & T. N. Postlethwaite (Eds.), *The international encyclopedia of education* (pp. 1643–1647). New York: Elsevier Sciences.
29. Garcia Coll, C., Crnic, K., Lamberty, G., Wasik, B. H., Jenkins, R., Garcia, H. V., & McAdoo, H. P. (1996). An integrative model for the study of developmental competencies in minority children. *Child Development, 67*(5), 1891–1914.
30. Coleman, J. S. (1961). *The adolescent society: The social life of the teenager and its Impact on Education*. Glencoe, IL: Free Press.

Chapter 2
The Relevance of the Social-Ecological Model and the Significance of Stratification

Abstract In Chap. 2, we establish the parameters of the theoretical framework that guides this book. We detail how diversity in disparities matter when utilizing the social-ecological framework. Under this theoretical framework, a youth's development occurs within a context of the system of relationships that form their social environments; however, we highlight how it is important to consider the significance of social stratification and inequality when investigating the connections between social environment and youth development.

Keywords Social-ecological model · Social stratification · School environment · School climate

Introduction

In this chapter, we argue that understanding social inequality and social stratification matters when understanding bullying within the social-ecological context. *Social stratification* is referred to as a process by which social inequalities are prevalent and maintained by differentiating an individual based upon occupation, income, or social status, or derived *power* [1]. One salient component of bullying is the *power imbalance* that exists between the perpetrator (or a group of perpetrators) and the victim. As highlighted by Dan Olweus, a pioneering researcher on school bullying, "It must be stressed that the term bullying is not (or should not be) used when two students of approximately the same strength (physical or psychological) are fighting or quarreling. To use the term bullying, there should be an imbalance in strength (an asymmetric power relationship): The student who is exposed to the negative actions has difficulty defending him/herself and is somewhat helpless against the student or students who harass" [2, p. 10].

Scholars have long argued that school bullying is a phenomenon that is influenced or inhibited by multiple contexts, including home, school, peer group, neighborhood, and society. Moreover, each subsystem depends on the contextual nature

A. A. Peguero, J. S. Hong, *School Bullying*, Springer Series on Child and Family Studies, https://doi.org/10.1007/978-3-030-64367-6_2

of a youth's life. A plethora of empirical research has utilized Bronfenbrenner's [3] seminal ecological systems framework to investigate multiple level factors that are related to school bullying within the family, school, and neighborhood contexts. Garcia Coll and colleagues [4] extended Bronfenbrenner's [3] social-ecological approach by proposing that when investigating the role of the social environment of youth who are marginalized and at risk of bullying involvement, it is important to understand that bullying may be shaped by (1) social position (e.g., race, gender), (2) social stratification (e.g., biased treatment), (3) promoting or inhibiting environments (e.g., school), (4) adaptive culture and current demands (e.g., assimilation or acculturation), (5) youth characteristics (e.g., psychological characteristics), and (6) family (e.g., structure, functioning).

Social Position

Perpetrators of bullying bully others to uphold their social position in school [5]. As Smith and Sharp [6] had argued, bullying is "systematic abuse of power," which not only is carried out for personal gain but also for the purpose of upholding emotions and status that accompany humiliating the victim. According to one study, achieving social status motivates one to engage in bullying but also increases the severity of the consequences of bullying [7]. Not surprisingly, students who are vulnerable physically or socially are highly likely to be victimized [7]. Also, an adolescent's social position, based on race/ethnicity and gender, can increase or decrease his or her risk of school bullying involvement. Being of a racial and ethnic minority can be perceived as a liability in U.S. schools, where bullying and harassment are all too frequent. The goal of the U.S. school systems has been to ensure that all students achieve educational success, which would translate into skills in the real world. However, due to inequality, minority students might have some difficulties in accessing and following formal education. Minority students are frequently bullied or singled out by their peers in school because of their physical traits, cultural background, limited English ability (for foreign-born students) [8, 9]. Foreign-born students are perceived to be of lower status, and as a result, they are at a higher risk of being bullied than their U.S.-born peers [8]. Concerning *gender*, males are regarded as more aggressive sex, and they are involved in bullying more frequently than females, as numerous research has shown [10]. Males are generally bigger and stronger than females physically, and they are more likely to seek social status and dominance and are more likely to participate in aggressive acts than females [11]. Males who are perceived to be weak or perceived as not fitting the hetero-normative masculine norms occupy lower social positions, which can elevate the likelihood of being bullied and picked on by stronger, more popular boys [see 12]. Also, in terms of bullying, males are more likely than females to perceive fighting to be an appropriate response when they feel disrespected [12]. Also, as cited in Kimmel [13], "[t]here are times when every boy must defend his own rights if he is not to become a coward, and lose the road to independence and true manhood" (p. 161). Researchers over the years, however, have also documented that girls are frequently engaged in another type of aggression, *relational aggression*, in which gossiping, spreading rumors, and excluding a target from social circles are typically involved [see [11]] to maintain dominance. However, other, more recent studies have also reported no gender differences in bullying involvement [e.g., 10].

Social Stratification

According to sociologists, *social stratification* is an unequal distribution of resources in society (income, wealth, occupation, education) [1]. Social stratification and poverty can affect the context in which youth interact and where bullying occurs [14]. There are two interrelated ways in which social stratification might operate to increase children's and adolescents' risk of bullying [15]. First, inequalities in income, education, or norms related to ethnicity, gender, and sexuality can shape school and community environments and the interpersonal relations that are in these environments, which can render some children vulnerable to victimization. Some children are at a heightened risk of being victims of bullying because they are labeled as different from other children or because they are targets of stigma, which is directed toward certain social groups [15]. Empirical evidence has shown that adolescents of lower social status are bullied and marginalized in school at a higher rate than their peers of higher social status [e.g., 16]. In an international survey of 162,305 students (ages 11, 13, and 15) in 35 countries, Due et al. [16] reported that youth from low-income families reported a higher prevalence of bullying victimization than those of higher-income families. The researchers concluded that there exist socioeconomic inequalities in bullying exposure among adolescents, which leaves youth of socioeconomic disadvantage at higher risk of victimization. Impoverished children's lack of resources may set them apart from their peers, in terms of materials: for example, clothing and money. A report by the Children's Society [17] found that children living in low-income families felt embarrassed because their families were unable to afford school costs, and 25% said this they were bullied as a result. Moreover, children of lower social status are likely to have family problems, such as coming from a single-parent household, having an incarcerated parent, or coming from foster care, which can subject them to taunting, teasing, and bullying by their classmates and peers.

Promoting or Inhibiting Environments

An adolescent's social environments, including home, school, and neighborhood, and how they may contribute to bullying and peer victimization has been researched widely. Because of the prevailing social stratification, certain environments can increase the risk while others can reduce the risk of bullying. In terms of families, certain family characteristics, such as single-parent households, lower parental educational attainment, low socioeconomic status, and parental incarceration are shown to be positively related to becoming a target or participant of bullying [10, 18]. Children growing up in such households are probably predisposed to violence exposure in the family and maltreatment, which can increase victimization risk outside of the home [10, 19]. Schools, which are important institutions where children spend a great deal of their time with peers, is an important context for understanding children's bullying involvement. A school climate that is characterized by having low resources, violence, and high criminal activities can expose children to aggressive peer interactions and can reinforce cultural norms supportive of violence [see 20]. Recognizing the importance of the school climate, several anti-bullying programs have targeted the entire school (i.e., "whole-school") to promote support from staff and peers [e.g., 21]. Compared to research on the link between home and school environments and bullying, studies exploring neighborhood environment and youths' involvement in bullying are limited. Like schools, neighborhoods that are characterized as low resourced and crime-prone can increase the development of aggressive and bullying behaviors in children and adolescents [22]. Children living in stratified and low-resourced neighborhoods may feel a sense of hopelessness because of adult authorities due to the absence of adult authorities (absence of capable guardians) [23]. As a consequence, these children are vulnerable to victimization because they are "suitable targets" of motivated offenders (opportunities) [23]. Also, these children are likely to have greater opportunities to exhibit aggressive behavior and violent tendencies to reduce the risk of victimization [24].

Adaptive Culture and Current Demands

Recent scholarships on bullying, particularly those focusing on immigration and bullying, have explored the role of cultural adaptation, including assimilation and acculturation. Extant research, however, has produced mixed findings. Pottie and colleagues' [8] study using a nationally representative sample of adolescents reported that immigrant youth are more likely to become victims of bullying than their native-born peers. Another study, which included a nationally representative sample of adolescents, found that immigrant youth are more likely to experience bullying victimization than native-born youth [25]. Other studies, report the lower likelihood of bullying among first-generation adolescents than their U.S.-born peers who tend to be more assimilated to the mainstream society [26, 27], although first-generation adolescents are more likely to report being afraid of going to the school they attend [27]. Also, Pottie and colleagues' [8] study showed that first-generation adolescents are more at risk of bullying victimization than are third-generation adolescents. Immigrant children are less likely to misbehave in school and are more likely to academically outperform their assimilated, native-born peers [28–30]. It is conceivable that for some first-generation immigrants, they are less likely to be engaged in misbehavior because they have a lot to lose (e.g., fear of deportation), and avoiding legal entanglement is a high priority [31]. Consequently, parents of first-generation immigrant children tend to teach their children the importance of "playing by the rules," even though these deterrent and motivational effects may subside for the more assimilated immigrants [31]. However, foreign-born adolescents may also be targeted by their mainstream and assimilated peers. In the daily experiences of immigrant children, English proficiency is intricately linked to many student experiences in U.S. schools. Immigrant children with heavy accents and limited English-speaking proficiency are frequently subjected to discrimination, teasing, harassment, and bullying by their classmates, peers, teachers, and school administrators [32], which impede school access and ability to participate in certain programs and activities [32].

Youth Characteristics

Individual characteristics of children, particularly certain psychological characteristics such as internalizing problems (e.g., depression, anxiety, low self-esteem), and low empathy are risk markers for children's involvement in bullying in schools. Children and adolescents who are depressed and exhibit anxiety and low self-esteem are especially vulnerable to victimization [33]. They are perceived by their peers as being psychologically weak and hold low social standing amongst their peers [see 34]. Juvonen and colleagues' [34] study, which was derived from a community sample of Latino and African American sixth-graders in eleven schools, found that youth identified as bullies were psychologically strongest and held high social position among their peers. On the other hand, victims were found to be emotionally distressed and socially alienated. Because of low social standing, depressed and anxious children are perceived by their peers to be lacking confidence and are unlikely to retaliate when they are bullied by their peers [35]. Additionally, a significant amount of research studies also investigated the association between low empathy and bullying participation, and most of these findings showed that low empathy predicted bullying behavior [36–38]. Children, particularly adolescents, who show low levels of empathy are likely to be involved with antisocial and deviant peer groups who may engage in reckless and delinquent behaviors, which may also include peer aggression. It is also plausible that youth who display low levels of empathy is likely to be rejected, victimized, and marginalized by their mainstream peer groups, as they are often perceived as being antisocial. However, one study, which examined the linkage between affective and cognitive empathy and bullying involvement in elementary and middle school students found a positive relationship between affective empathy and defending behavior among males with high social status [39]. The complex association between empathy and bullying is evident as adolescents may struggle between the desire to "fit in" and the desire to not hurt others.

Family

Family structure and functioning are crucial to the development of children's relationships and socialization in school and the neighborhood; therefore, it appears that parents are influential in their children's participation in, or exposure to bullying [40]. Numerous theories, such as attachment theory to social learning theory and family systems theory provide explanations as to how the family might influence on children's risk of bullying and peer victimization [40]. According to the attachment theory, the quality of attachment between the child and primary caregivers shapes a child's interpersonal relationships with others, such as friends, peers, and teachers [41]. The social learning theory proposes that children develop (aggressive or violent) behaviors by observing and role modeling [41]. Bowen's family systems theory argues that an individual child cannot be understood individually; rather, they must be understood as a part of their family [42]. According to the family systems theory, because the family is an emotional unit, family dynamics can shed light on the quality of peer relations among children and adolescents. As detailed in Chap. 3, certain characteristics of the family, such as low level of parental involvement, a lack of parental monitoring, authoritarian parenting style, and maltreatment are just some of the several family-level predictors that were considered in research on bullying [10]. These predictors may be influenced by the existing social stratification in society. It is no surprise that social inequality and lack of resources, including low family income and low educational attainment of parents can seriously undermine the lack of bonding and attachment between a parent and a child, as well as parenting style, thus contributing to children's bullying involvement.

Complexities

The relevance of macrosystem level factors, such as social stratification in understanding children's bullying and peer victimization has been seriously understudied. However, as Bronfenbrenner [3] proposed, "[t]he macrosystem refers to the overarching institutional patterns of the culture or subculture, such as the economic, social, educational, legal, and political systems [e.g., social stratification], of which micro-, meso-, and exosystems are the concrete manifestations" [p. 515]. In other words, the influences of the antecedents of bullying at the multiple levels—individual characteristics, family structure, peer group, school, and neighborhood climates, and cultural adaptation can be shaped by social stratification that exists in broader society. This is particularly important when understanding how school bullying is experienced by oppressed and historically marginalized social groups, including racial and ethnic minorities, immigrants, gender and sexual minorities, and those with physical, emotional, and learning disabilities. Over the past several decades, the demographic characteristics of the U.S. population, which was previously perceived to be white and middle class, speaking English only, and living in a nuclear family, have changed dramatically [43]. Also, the future is likely to reflect the even greater change; for example, it is predicted that whites will account for approximately 10% of new entrants in the U.S. workforce, and minority and immigrant males, along with women are likely to account for over half of the growth in employment in U.S. labor force [43]. Despite the changing population trends, children and adolescents of minoritized social groups are growing populations. However, these children frequently are still subjected to bullying, teasing, ridicule, taunting, and harassment due to actual or perceived differences and their presumed inability to conform to the mainstream school districts in the United States. To better understand the underlying mechanisms of children's bullying, which can later evolve into more effective prevention and intervention strategies, it would be useful to explore the experiences of these children in school bullying. In addition to identifying new variables, it would be worthwhile to explore how societal, community, institutional, peer, and individual contexts might converge to reinforce or inhibit school bullying and victimization among diverse groups of children who are increasingly representing the student demographics in the United States.

Conclusion

This chapter is consistent with Garcia Coll and colleagues' [4] argument that diverse children's bullying and peer victimization in U.S. schools must take into account (1) social position, (2) social stratification, (3) promoting or inhibiting environments, (4) adaptive culture and current demands, (5) youth characteristics, and (6) family. We would like to remind the readers that social stratification can and does intersect with a variety of social identities, including race and ethnicity, immigrant status, gender, sexual orientation, gender identity, gender expression, and disabilities, any of which can heighten or reduce school bullying.

References

1. Beeghley, L. (2008). *The structure of social stratification in the United States*. New York: Taylor & Francis.
2. Olweus, D. (1993). *Bullying at school: What we know and what we can do*. Oxford, UK: Blackwell Publishers.
3. Bronfenbrenner, U. (1979). *The ecology of human development: Experiments by nature and design*. Cambridge, MA: Harvard University Press.
4. Garcia Coll, C., Crnic, K., Lamberty, G., Wasik, B. H., Jenkins, R., Garcia, H. V., & McAdoo, H. P. (1996). An integrative model for the study of developmental competencies in minority children. *Child Development, 67*(5), 1891–1914.
5. Stuart-Cassel, V., Terzian, M., & Bradshaw, C. (2013). *Social bullying: Correlates, consequences, and prevention. In Brief.* National Center on Safe Supportive Learning Environments.

6. Sharp, S., & Smith, P. (1994). *School bullying: Insights and perspectives*. London, UK: Routledge.
7. Faris, R., & Felmlee, D. (2014). Casualties of social combat: School networks of peer victimization and their consequences. *American Sociological Review, 79*(2), 228–257.
8. Pottie, K., Dahal, G., Georgiades, K., Premji, K., & Hassan, G. (2015). Do first generation immigrant adolescents face higher rates of bullying, violence and suicidal behaviours than do third generation and native born? *Journal of Immigrant and Minority Health, 17*(5), 1557–1566.
9. Qin, D. B., Way, N., & Rana, M. (2008). The "model minority" and their discontent: Examining peer discrimination and harassment of Chinese American immigrant youth. *New Directions for Child and Adolescent Development, 2008*(121), 27–42.
10. Hong, J. S., & Espelage, D. L. (2012). A review of research on bullying and peer victimization in school: An ecological system analysis. *Aggression and Violent Behavior, 17*(4), 311–322.
11. Espelage, D. L., & Swearer, S. M. (2003). Research on school bullying and victimization: What have we learned and where do we go from here? *School Psychology Review, 32*(3), 365–383.
12. Kimmel, M. S., & Mahler, M. (2003). Adolescent masculinity, homophobia, and violence: Random school shootings, 1982-2001. *American Behavioral Scientist, 46*(10), 1439–1458.
13. Kimmel, M. S. (1996). *Manhood in America: A cultural history*. New York: Free Press.
14. Elgar, F. J., Craig, W., Boyce, W., Morgan, A., & Vella-Zarb, R. (2009). Income inequality and school bullying: Multilevel study of adolescents in 37 countries. *Journal of Adolescent Health, 45*(4), 351–359.
15. Pells, K., Portela, M. J. O., Revollo, P. E., et al. (2016). *Experiences of peer bullying among adolescents and associated effects on young adult outcomes: Longitudinal evidence from Ethiopia, India, Peru and Viet Nam*. UN.
16. Due, P., Merlo, J., Harel-Fisch, Y., Damsgaard, M. T., soc, M. scient, Holstein, B. E., et al. (2009). Socioeconomic inequality in exposure to bullying during adolescence: A comparative, cross-sectional, multilevel study in 35 countries. American Journal of Public Health, 99(5), 907–914.
17. Children's Society. (2014). At what cost exposing the impact of poverty on school life—full report. *The Children's Society*. Retrieved August 10, 2020, from https://www.childrenssociety.org.uk/what-we-do/resources-and-publications/publications-library/at-what-cost-exposing-the-impact-of-poverty-on-school-life-full-report
18. Ttofi, M. M., & Farrington, D. P. (2011). Effectiveness of school-based programs to reduce bullying: A systematic and meta-analytic review. *Journal of Experimental Criminology, 7*(1), 27–56.
19. Shields, A., & Cicchetti, D. (2001). Parental maltreatment and emotion dysregulation as risk factors for bullying and victimization in middle childhood. *Journal of Clinical Child Psychology, 30*(3), 349–363.
20. Unnever, J. D., & Cornell, D. G. (2003). The culture of bullying in middle school. *Journal of School Violence, 2*(2), 5–27.
21. Eliot, M., Cornell, D., Gregory, A., & Fan, X. (2010). Supportive school climate and student willingness to seek help for bullying and threats of violence. *Journal of School Psychology, 48*(6), 533–553.
22. Low, S., & Espelage, D. (2014). Conduits from community violence exposure to peer aggression and victimization: Contributions of parental monitoring, impulsivity, and deviancy. *Journal of Counseling Psychology, 61*(2), 221.
23. Felson, M., & Cohen, L. E. (1980). Human ecology and crime: A routine activity approach. *Human Ecology, 8*(4), 389–406.
24. Anderson, E. (1999). *Code of the street: Decency, violence, and the moral life of the inner city*. New York: Norton.

25. Maynard, B. R., Vaughn, M. G., Salas-Wright, C. P., & Vaughn, S. (2016). Bullying victimization among school-aged immigrant youth in the United States. *Journal of Adolescent Health, 58*(3), 337–344.
26. Peguero, A. A. (2008). Is immigrant status relevant in school violence research? An analysis with Latino students. *Journal of School Health, 78*(7), 397–404.
27. Peguero, A. A. (2009). Victimizing the children of immigrants: Latino and Asian American student victimization. *Youth & Society, 41*(2), 186–208.
28. Peguero, A. A. (2012). Schools, bullying, and inequality: Intersecting factors and complexities with the stratification of youth victimization at school. *Sociology Compass, 6*(5), 402–412.
29. Peguero, A. A., Bondy, J. M., & Hong, J. S. (2017). Social bonds across immigrant generations: Bonding to school and examining the relevance of assimilation. *Youth & Society, 49*(6), 733–754.
30. Peguero, A. A., & Shekarkhar, Z. (2011). Latino/a student misbehavior and school punishment. *Hispanic Journal of Behavioral Sciences, 33*(1), 54–70.
31. Vaughn, M. G., Salas-Wright, C. P., Maynard, B. R., Qian, Z., Terzis, L., Kusow, A. M., & DeLisi, M. (2014). Criminal epidemiology and the immigrant paradox: Intergenerational discontinuity in violence and antisocial behavior among immigrants. *Journal of Criminal Justice, 42*(6), 483–490.
32. Peguero, A. A. (2008). The victimization and vulnerabilities of immigrant children: The importance of English proficiency. Agenda for social justice*:* Solutions, 1–7.
33. Schwartz, D., McFadyen-Ketchum, S., Dodge, K. A., Pettit, G. S., & Bates, J. E. (1999). Early behavior problems as a predictor of later peer group victimization: Moderators and mediators in the pathways of social risk. *Journal of Abnormal Child Psychology, 27*(3), 191–201.
34. Juvonen, J., Graham, S., & Schuster, M. A. (2003). Bullying among young adolescents: The strong, the weak, and the troubled. *Pediatrics, 112*(6), 1231–1237.
35. Fekkes, M., Pijpers, F. I., & Verloove-Vanhorick, S. P. (2005). Bullying: Who does what, when and where? Involvement of children, teachers and parents in bullying behavior. *Health Education Research, 20*(1), 81–91.
36. Endresen, I. M., & Olweus, D. (2001). Self-reported empathy in Norwegian adolescents: Sex differences, age trends, and relationship to bullying. In *Constructive & destructive behavior: Implications for family, school, & society*. Washington, DC: American Psychological Association.
37. Jolliffe, D., & Farrington, D. P. (2006). Examining the relationship between low empathy and bullying. Aggressive Behavior. *Official Journal of the International Society for Research on Aggression, 32*(6), 540–550.
38. Jolliffe, D., & Farrington, D. P. (2011). Is low empathy related to bullying after controlling for individual and social background variables? *Journal of Adolescence, 34*(1), 59–71.
39. Caravita, S. C., Di Blasio, P., & Salmivalli, C. (2009). Unique and interactive effects of empathy and social status on involvement in bullying. *Social Development, 18*(1), 140–163.
40. Holt, M. K., Kaufman Kantor, G., & Finkelhor, D. (2008). Parent/child concordance about bullying involvement and family characteristics related to bullying and peer victimization. *Journal of School Violence, 8*(1), 42–63.
41. Monks, C. P., Smith, P. K., Naylor, P., Barter, C., Ireland, J. L., & Coyne, I. (2009). Bullying in different contexts: Commonalities, differences and the role of theory. *Aggression and Violent Behavior, 14*(2), 146–156.
42. Bowen, M. (1993). *Family therapy in clinical practice*. Jason Aronson.
43. Appleby, G. A., Colon, E., & Hamilton, J. (2011). *Diversity, oppression, and social functioning: Person-in-environment assessment and intervention*. Allyn & Bacon.

Chapter 3
Status Matters: How Socioeconomic and Social Statuses Are Associated with Bullying

Abstract In Chap. 3, we discuss how socioeconomic and social statuses are associated with bullying victimization. Low socioeconomic status, particularly living in poverty, is a risk factor for violence exposure in low-income communities and the schools that are embedded within them. In general, impoverished youth are significantly more likely to be exposed to peer violence and bullying victimization in school and are also likely to identify with a culture of violence. We also discuss how research has consistently found that social groups or statuses in school are important about experiences, expectations, and interactions. A youth's social status in school can be linked to his or her likelihood of being bullied. We also demonstrate how students with low social acceptance, high social rejection, or those who are labeled as nonaggressive are more likely to be victimized in school.

Keywords Socioeconomic status · Social status · Friendships · Social networks · Bystanders

Introduction

In this chapter, we explore how socioeconomic and social statuses are relevant to school bullying. Most school bullying research has focused on the differential patterns of victimization between poor and affluent youth. Research, however, suggests significant differences in the likelihood of victimization of poor students as well as how bullying victimization is defined by youth themselves. The same could also be said with social status. In general, social status is often associated with popularity and friendships or social networks. Research suggests that a student's popularity and friendships or social networks can be linked to the likelihood of bullying victimization and aggression that student experiences at school. We first discuss how socioeconomic status is related to being victimized while in U.S. schools. We then present how characteristics correlated to social status can influence the likelihood of school bullying victimization. We then discuss how socioeconomic and social

A. A. Peguero, J. S. Hong, *School Bullying*, Springer Series on Child and Family Studies, https://doi.org/10.1007/978-3-030-64367-6_3

statuses should be considered in the phenomenon of victimization at school through a social-ecological framework. In the final section of this chapter, we highlight the complexities associated with socioeconomic and social statuses with school bullying and victimization.

Socioeconomic Status

First and foremost, it is important to define socioeconomic status. The aggregate concept of the socioeconomic status is comprised of resource-based (i.e., material and social resources) and prestige-based (i.e., individual's rank or status) indicators of social and economic position, which is measured across societal levels (individual, household, and neighborhood) and at different periods. Moreover, socioeconomic status is often assessed through individual measures, such as education, income, or occupation, but also through composite measures that combine or assign weights to various socioeconomic aspects to provide a total index of socioeconomic level. Even though there is no set standard measure of socioeconomic status; indicators are used to measure specific aspects of social stratification, including poverty and affluence [1–4].

There are three broad ways socioeconomic status can contribute to youth violence and school bullying victimization. First, research evidence demonstrates that living in neighborhoods with high concentrations of poverty increases children's risks for social-psychological maladjustment (e.g., aggression, limited social skills) and exposure to youth interpersonal violence [5–7]. Second, it is evident that concentrated poverty at the school-level is associated with elevated levels of social-psychological maladjustment, poor conflict-resolution skills, and interpersonal violence among students [5–7]. Additionally, school-level poverty, often measured at the proportion of children eligible for free or reduced lunch, is associated with students' risk for being aggressive, less socially skilled, thereby increasing students' risks for being bullied or victimized [5–7]. Third, as noted in the introductory chapter, the role of power in bullying is important, and thus socioeconomic status can play an important role in the source of tension or conflict between students [5–7].

In 2013, for the first time since the 1970s, a majority of U.S. public school students come from low-income families [8]. Considering the relationship between socioeconomic status and bullying victimization, the increasing trend of socioeconomic inequality in the United States could have serious implications for individual student risk of being bullied as well as the overall rate of bullying occurring across U.S. schools. To be clear, as we will discuss in more detail later in this chapter, we are not indicating that poor or affluent students are more likely to be a bully or be victimized. We are suggesting is that the social-ecology of youth residing and attending school in poor or affluent communities is contributing to the likelihood of a student being a victim of bullying as well as the degree of the consequence of victimization.

Social Status

Since Coleman's [9] *The Adolescent Society*, researchers repeatedly find that social statuses and associated stereotypes in high school are defining behavioral norms and expectations. Social statuses such as "preppies or rich kids," "geeks or nerds," "jocks or athletes," and so forth remain meaningful today in schools as they were five decades ago when Coleman first reported their significance in adolescent school experiences [10–14]. Research demonstrates that more popular students are argued to be more insulated from being bullied and victimized at school because offenders or bullies face a possibility of social sanctions from other students as well as disciplinary action from teachers, administrators, or security [10–14]. It is conceptually argued that popular students are perceived and socially constructed as more valuable, and the injury or victimization of popular students as more serious [10–14]. To that end, the counter-narrative is also supported by the research.

Less popular students or those who are positioned lower in the social status hierarchy within schools garner less attention from fellow students, teachers, and staff [10–14]. Moreover, classmates often do not want to be associated with students who are often victimized and lower in the social hierarchy for fear of losing their social status positioning [10–14]. As such, victimization and peer rejection, as well as victimization and low perceived popularity, are likely to reinforce each other over time. In other words, a student's position in the social status hierarchy can be associated with vulnerability or insulation from victimization or being bullied at school for a long period. Thus, popularity can be perceived as a form of capital or value that warrants protection, which can certainly complicate interpersonal relationships for want to remain popular.

Recent studies have revealed that popular students often engage in bullying as a means to remain popular and secure their position in the social status hierarchy [10–14]. Bullies are often disliked by their peers but there is a trend of recent studies that popular students are engaging in bullying as means to sustain and maintain their social status as well as broaden their social authority over other students [10–12, 14]. Salmivalli [15] reports that bullies often impose their aggressive or dominant behavior because of having "high status and a powerful, dominant position in the peer group" [p. 113]. Also, students can seek to increase or maintain a powerful social status position in the group by bullying because their powerful social position allows them to bully classmates [10–14]. It is also believed that bystander students who witness bullying from a popular student might learn from the social bullying event at school and replicate the bullying behavior to increase their social standing by appearing more like the person in power, that is, the bully [16]. Once again, as we will discuss in more detail later in this chapter, we are not arguing that popular students are going to bully and that unpopular students will be bullied; however, we do suggest that the socio-ecological framework of the social and cultural definitions, values, and behaviors associated with bullying and what is tolerated or expected from popular students is critical toward understanding the complexities linked to the relationship between social status and school bullying.

Friendships, Social Networks, and Bystanders

School friendships offer support, affection, and a sense of school belonging and belief in the educational process, promote pro-social experiences and strong interpersonal relationships within the school, and potentially foster a belief that school is a safe and healthy learning environment [11, 12, 17]. As for bullying, having an increased number of friends at school could be a protective factor against being victimized [11, 12, 17]; however, there are some caveats. For instance, having supportive, empathetic, and caring friends could shield against being bullied, but having aggressive friends could result in an increased chance of being victimized [11, 12, 17]. There are a complex school friendship and victimization dynamic among bullied students. It is argued that victimized children often befriend other victimized children while non-victimized children avoid befriending victimized peers and prefer to affiliate with other non-victimized children [11, 12, 17]. Nevertheless, students who have close and strong friendships can minimize or ameliorate the detrimental effects that being bullied can have.

There is a broad social notion that people often "get ahead" by making social or interpersonal connections with many different people as well as being pleasant and fostering those social or interpersonal relationships, because being sociable and having "networks" translates into prestige, opportunities, and resources. This notion has become applicable in social network analyses of aggression and bullying within schools. Broadly, there two aspects of social networks: centralization and density. Centralization refers to whether social network ties have a more hierarchical or more egalitarian pattern. Carolan [18, p. 107] argues, "networks that are centralized, regardless of their density, are ones in which only a small and exclusive set of actors hold positions of power and control. Decentralized networks, conversely, are those in which power and control are diffuse and spread over a number of actors." Egalitarian social networks within the school could have more positive social interactions such as increased cooperation, pro-social behavior, less peer rejection, decreased likelihood of being victimized or bullied [11, 19]. On the contrary, hierarchical social networks within a school are associated with increased hostility, aggression, bullying, and diminished cohesion [11, 19]. In school bullying research dense social networks are often measured as student peers nominate or acknowledge a particular student as a friend [11, 19]. In other words, the more student classmates denote a particular student as a friend, the denser the social network, and the less likely that student will be bullied [19]. However, the fewer student classmates denote a particular student as a friend, the less dense the social network, that student will have an increased likelihood of being bullied [19].

There is research that highlights the role of bystanders in school bullying. Twemlow, Fonagy, and Sacco [20] defined a bystander as an individual who does not participate in bullying incidents as either the bully or victim. The bystander may actively intervene to deter the bullying, encourage the bully to continue, or view bullying passively [21–23]. There are three general categories of bystanders associated with school bullying: reinforcing, passive, and defending. Reinforcing bystanders are students who affirm or encourage the bully socially through laughing, making emboldening comments, or serving as an approving audience; moreover, research suggests that student reinforcers are associated with increased occurrences of bullying within a school [21–23]. Passive bystanders are students who witness bullying but take no action; additionally, it also appears that passive student reinforcers can also contribute to increased bullying incidents within a school [21–23]. Defending bystanders are students who actively seek to stop bullies, help victims, and/or alert an adult of bullying occurring; furthermore, student defenders are linked to decreased bullying rates within a school [21–23]. With this noted, there are complexities associated with understanding bystanders, such as a particular student may play a different role at different times depending on the friendships, the social network, or other factors [21–23]. It is conceptualized that, for the bully, laughter is a form of encouragement, and sometimes just having a captivated student audience could be interpreted as valued and acceptable behavior by the bully. Without such social affirmation, bullies may be far less likely to engage in aggressive or bullying behavior [21–23]. Student victims who have at least one defender may also experience less anxiety and depression than those who have no defenders [21–23].

Social-Ecological Framework

In this section, we present the significance of socioeconomic and social statuses in the context of bullying victimization through a social-ecological framework. Although we will not specifically illustrate how societal, community, institutional, group, and individual status relates to socioeconomic and social statuses, we will provide a general overview. Then, we will follow up with a discussion of the complexities associated with linking bullying victimization, socioeconomic and social statuses, and the social-ecological framework.

Societal

At the societal level, educational and economic inequalities have indirect and direct implications toward schools and their students being vulnerable to violence as well as having the capabilities or resources to respond and address bullying. This societal-level highlights the historical, structural, systemic, and overarching economic disparities in the U.S. are associated with school violence, victimization, and bullying.

All stratification systems require "a social structure that divides people into categories" [24, p. 242]. Educational systems are among the most important such structures in contemporary societies [1, 2, 24]. It is argued that educational categories structure the competition for positions in stratified societies and, in the process, an influence which individuals attain which social locations [1, 2, 24]. Therefore, schools, as well as stratified educational categories, shape the inequality structure of the societies in which they operate. Educational inequality in the U.S. is historic and persistent with serious implications for the violence and safety of students across schools. Schools are a fundamental mechanism that determines which positions specific students to occupy in unequal societies, as well as in determining and legitimating disparities between students within educational hierarchies along which reproduce social inequalities [1, 2, 24].

There is a long history of research demonstrating that schools reflect the communities to which they serve which often reflects the economic resources available to that school [1, 24, 25]. The allocation of educational resources as well as the federal, state, county, district, and local political decisions associated are argued to contribute to educational inequality [1, 24, 25]. Often, when school district boundaries or admission eligibility are established, these societal lines are reflective socioeconomic status which produces the quantity and quality of educational resources and academic prestige vary across schools [1, 24, 25]. In turn, school resource disparities have been associated with how many school safety programs can implement and how effective and efficient these programs are with reducing bullying and victimization [5, 13, 26]. Even though school administration and staff training, regular program evaluations, prosocial activities, performance management, and the like are associated with ameliorating violence and bullying at schools, the resources often needed to sustain school safety programs are more accessible at more affluent schools than disadvantaged schools [5, 13, 26].

There is a growing recognition that bullying is a serious problem that impels federal, state, county, district, and local educational policymakers and officials to consider what is the best way to implement school policies that ensures the safety of student [5, 25–27]. Moreover, many state legislators have become interested in passing laws to influence the development of school-based violence and anti-bullying prevention policies. However, bullying and school violence prevention programs, in general, have not considered the difference between schools located in affluent or middle-class schools as opposed to disadvantaged schools [5, 13, 26, 28]. The prevalence of bullying and aggressive behavior in disadvantaged states, counties, and local school districts are often faced with a wide array of economic barriers and hurdles to provide healthy and safe school environments for their students despite unfunded federal and state mandates to address violence and bullying within schools [5, 13, 26, 28].

Community

Disadvantaged and violent community environments could contribute to being victimized at school because researchers consistently find community resources and/or socioeconomic influences on youth outcomes, including physical inactivity, obesity, school achievement, perceived health status, mental health, victimization, and behavioral problems [6, 29, 30]. The impact of adverse community conditions, particularly neighborhood deprivation, on health and behavioral outcomes has been shown to persist even after controlling for parental socioeconomic status.

A community "disorder" or "incivilities" thesis [6, 29, 31, 32] suggests that the conditions of an individual's surroundings can be a significant correlate toward understanding their behavior, exposure to violence, and vulnerability to being victimized. In essence, the disorder thesis argues that deteriorating physical and social conditions of a community (i.e., broken windows) could facilitate increases in crime, delinquency, and youth victimization [6, 29, 31, 32]. The process from disorder to violence and victimization could occur because disorder and/or incivility are presumed to lead to fear among individuals; this fear, in turn, is posited to prompt individual withdrawal, leaving the area vulnerable to more serious criminal invasion [6, 29, 31, 32]. Therefore, the disorder and/or incivilities thesis conceptualizes a downward spiral of disorder, fear, withdrawal, and criminal or delinquent expansion [6, 29, 31, 32].

Prior research has demonstrated that youth often feel unsafe as well as get victimized, harassed, and bullied to and from school. Various aspects of bullying (physical, social, and verbal) can reinforce fear and perceived unsafety among students who are going to or from their school [33–35]. It also appears that there is a higher reported risk by students in disadvantaged communities. Many disadvantaged and low-resourced communities are situated in more densely populated urban areas, and youth in these areas are highly likely to walk to and from school than their suburban and rural student counterparts [33–35]. As a result, there is emerging research that also associates student avoidance and fear with disadvantaged community environments.

Institutional

At the institutional level, school level poverty, lack of resources, and faculty and staff turnover can have serious implications and cause barriers to practices or processes which may be associated with students' safety and victimization. It is argued that there is a strong relationship between disadvantaged and disorganized schools, particularly those in urban areas [31, 32, 36]. Research has suggested that higher levels of violence, misbehavior, bullying, and victimization in schools are often attributed to lack of school organization; in other words, disorganized schools tend to be unsuccessful in addressing problems of delinquency and violence as well as implementing prevention programs due to overburdened administrators, understaffing, and school climate [31, 36–38].

As we think about school-level processes, the social bond theory postulates that the strength of an adolescent's social bond to conventional individuals, society, and institutions (e.g., schools) will determine whether that adolescent will engage in conforming or delinquent behavior [39]. In essence, it has been argued that the stronger the social bonds among school participants and stakeholders (i.e., faculty, administrators, students, and parents), the lower the probability that delinquency, misbehavior, victimization, and bullying will occur at that school [27, 37, 40, 41]. For clarification, social bond to school consists of four elements: attachment, commitment, involvement, and belief. Attachment to school refers to the emotional connection between students and conventional others; the stronger the emotional connection to the school, the more likely the conventional others (such as teachers) will be to influence students' behavior away from delinquency, misbehavior, and bullying [27, 37, 40, 41]. Commitment to school refers to students' investment in conforming to society and the schools' expectations; the greater the investment, the less likely students will be to engage in delinquency, misbehavior, and bullying [27, 37, 40, 41]. Involvement in school extracurricular activities refers to the students' participation in conforming activities. Participation in conforming activities (e.g., sports, band, clubs, etc.) reduces the students' time available for engaging in delinquency, misbehavior, and bullying [27, 37, 40, 41]. Belief in the school refers to whether students accept the traditional value system of rules and incorporate them into their moral code; the stronger students' belief in the school rules, the less likely students will be to engage in delinquency, misbehavior, and bullying [27, 37, 40, 41]. In turn, there is evidence that school-based victimization is related to the strength of a student's social bond to school.

It is also clear, however, that schools that have limited economic and social resources face challenges in supporting and sustaining strong bonds at their schools. For each element of social bonds to school, there are serious barriers associated with disadvantaged and under-resourced schools. For attachment to school, because there are a significant administrator and teacher turnover at disadvantaged schools [27, 37, 40, 41], school inequality poses as a barrier to school attachment. For commitment to school, because research demonstrates that some disadvantaged schools have lower academic expectations, fewer educational opportunities, and unclear pathways toward scholastic progress and success [27, 37, 40, 41], these educational inequities reflect hurdles for school commitment for their students. For school involvement, since there are fewer extracurricular activities offered at poorer and under-resourced [27, 37, 40, 41], disadvantaged schools could pose limitations for students' school involvement. For belief in the school rules, because research demonstrates that discipline and punishment practices are argued to be nontransparent, unjust, and unfair at more disadvantaged schools [27, 40, 41], this school disparity can derail students' belief in the school rules. As a consequence, school-level practices and processes associated with students' bonding to their school way be impeded by the school's level of access to resources, which in turn may contribute to that school's bullying and victimization rates.

Group

School and classrooms are composed of student groups who share daily interactions and routines. This group-level shows friendships as well as the associated hierarchies linked to social status. The position of a student with that school, or classroom stratification, or hierarchy with social status and friendships may contribute to the risk of being a victim of bullying, harassment, and violence [10–12, 19]. A student's closest social circle of peers and their social identity could contribute to their odds of being bullied and victimized [10–12, 19].

A peer or group socioecological perspective stresses that schools are akin to a small society or social network in which students interact with, influence, and socialize one another [10–12, 19]. Interactions within and among student groups can take many forms, including frequent affiliation, joint participation in activities, as well as negative forms such as bullying victimization and antipathy. Friendships and social networks are fundamental to students' social development [10–12, 19]. Friendships and social networks can ameliorate negative outcomes that are associated with peer rejection and victimization [10–12, 19]. Inequalities associated with social status, friendship, and positioning of students within a school's hierarchy can contribute to a student's vulnerability to being victimized, harassed, and/or marginalized while at school [7, 10–12, 19]. Not all students have personal attributes or characteristics that can facilitate the opportunity to be popular. Researchers have often suggested that popular students, or students who have social network centrality, often have qualities such as socioeconomic affluence, attractiveness, athleticism, or charisma [7, 10–12, 19].

Researchers have argued that the relationship between aggression and social network centrality is reflective of two factors: (1) whether centrality might increase the capacity for aggressive behavior and (2) whether status is a primary motivation for engaging in aggressive behavior. Power-dependency theorists propose that social networks and social hierarchies create power imbalances by regulating the availability of alternative exchange partners [10–12]. Even if a student's network position is initially caused by personal qualities, the main actors are likely to be disproportionately affected by new nominations, not due to personal qualities, but under having already received many nominations [10–12]. In other words, the main actors or "popular" students have social lives that often do not rely on any single friend or group of friends, they can socially exclude others more easily than they can be socially excluded themselves [10–12]. This power connected with popular students affords them more leverage in each of their social networks and friendships impose dominance struggles [10–12].

Social status and friendships being associated with centrality indicate that power and influence are associated with that social position. Students who have a lot of power and influence in the social hierarchy have the potential to impose their interests [7, 10–12, 19]. Some have suggested that this "strong" position associated with social status can incorporate others (i.e., students, teachers, and staff) to reinforce or protect the social status hierarchy. For example, some have suggested that popular students often encourage their friends to harass, bully, marginalize, excuse, and/or isolate students [7, 10–12, 19]. Moreover, there is also research suggesting that administrators, teachers, staff, and security personnel often side with the "popular" students by disbelieving, or dismissing the reports of less popular student victims of violence and bullying [7, 10–12, 19].

Individual

Opportunity theory is often used to examine the insulating and risk factors that are associated with student victimization. Opportunity theory looks at the characteristics of both offenders and victims and/or the characteristics of the space where the offenders and victims are likely to have interactions at which is consequently linked to victimization [42]. It is also evident that adolescents in the U.S. experience increased risk of victimization, which can occur in schools where adolescents spend a great deal of time [13, 43–45]. Research has repeatedly demonstrated that opportunity theory is a highly relevant and effective theoretical framework that can explain the occurrence of student victimization [13, 43–45]; however, recent research findings also suggest distinctive nuances associated with socioeconomic and social statuses in the relationship between opportunity and student victimization.

Opportunity theory builds on routine activity and lifestyle theoretical frameworks which conceptualize factors that are associated with victimization. Routine activity theory highlights three necessary factors for crime to occur: (1) the presence and proximity of motivated offenders, (2) the presence of a suitable target, and (3) the absence of a capable guardian [13, 43–45]. Routine activity theory purports that victimization comes from the recurrent and prevalent activities that individuals are involved in daily which increases the odds that all three necessary factors will be present. Therefore, it is an individual's routines and activities that increase one's risk of victimization. Similarly, lifestyle theorists suggest that involvement in particular deviant groups or social activities may make a person more susceptible to victimization [13, 43–45]. Subsequently, researchers have integrated both routine activities and lifestyle theories to better understand the relationship between misbehavior and victimization. The principal logic driving the integration of these two theories concerning opportunity is centered on four factors that contribute to victimization—suitable targets, exposure, proximity to motivated offenders, and lack of guardianship [13, 43–45]. Inequalities associated with socioeconomic and social statuses have been found to moderate these elements of opportunity theory (i.e., target suitability, exposure, proximity to motivated offenders, and guardianship) that predict student misbehavior and victimization.

A *suitable target* refers to the perception of the potential victim as vulnerable by a motivated offender. Who is perceived as an "attractive student target" may be related to social status. For instance, involvement in certain academic activities (e.g., student government, band, and school newspaper) is linked to increased odds of being victimized at school; on the other hand, student-athletes are less likely to be victimized at school [13, 43–45]. The suggestion is that "smart" students are sometimes perceived as weak and are often victimized as a result, whereas athletes, who are perceived as being capable of protecting themselves, are not.

Exposure is the accessibility of individuals or objects to potential offenders at any moment or place [13, 43–45]. Involvement with delinquent peers, gangs, or individual misbehavior often results from increased exposure to victimization within and outside of school [13, 43–45]. Students who are frequently exposed to deviant and delinquent activities are at a heightened risk of being involved in those activities [13, 43–45]. Once youth participate in deviance, this behavior, in turn, increases their exposure to situations that are primed for victimization. For example, a student who is often socially excluded by mainstream peer groups may frequently be victimized because of their associations and interactions with deviant peers [13, 43–45]. Furthermore, as a student becomes more involved in a deviant lifestyle, the line between offender and victim grows difficult to distinguish, even within schools [13, 43–45].

Guardianship refers to the effectiveness of persons (e.g., security guards, law enforcement officers) or objects in preventing victimization from occurring, either by their presence alone or by some sort of direct or indirect action [13, 43–45]. In other words, the level of guardianship that is present within a particular context is argued to be a factor in the occurrence of victimization. Increasing guardianship and security has been a common response to student victimization; however, the implementation of increased school security measures varies between affluent and disadvantaged schools [4, 46–49]. More recently, there has been a growing trend of increasing school security in public school districts by increasing police presence and meting out punitive measures for student misbehaviors (e.g., zero-tolerance). An increasing number of public high school districts have law enforcement officers, armed security guards, metal detectors, surveillance cameras, and random searches [4, 46–49]. Researchers have argued that the number of school security measures tend to be significantly higher in poorer and disadvantaged schools [4, 46–49].

Proximity is conceptualized as a physical distance between potential targets of victimization and potential offenders, which is likely to lead to the occurrence of victimization [13, 43–45]. Schools with high levels of the social disorder are associated with an increased likelihood of victimization due to students' proximity to motivated offenders [13, 43–45]. Additionally, poorer urban and rural schools often have increased levels of misbehavior which increases the proximity to motivated offenders and increases the likelihood of victimization to occur [13, 43–45].

Complexities

Several complexities should be considered when trying to understand how socioeconomic and social statuses are associated with school bullying. As noted in the introductory chapter of this book, because the definition of bullying is complex and relative, school bullying policies may not address all forms of perceived bullying. In this context, the perception of violence, injury, and victimization is primarily based on adult definitions and understandings of bullying, which may lead to under- or over-monitoring of violent student behavior. In other words, school administrators, faculty, and staff interpretations may influence the utilization of bullying policies. Social and cultural complexities associated with socioeconomic status, social class, and social status are sometimes excluded from definitions of bullying and are therefore not addressed by bullying policies. For instance, there are reports of schools underutilizing bullying definitions that include tensions or conflict between poor and affluent students within a school for fear of the perception that parents and community will interpret this action as supportive of privilege and class conflict or biases [5, 7, 50]. Further, there is a clear socioeconomic gap between how bullying is defined, identified, and addressed by privileged schools as opposed to disadvantaged schools as well as a variety of socioeconomic and social statuses among the student body within a school, complicating how bullies and bullying victims are identified. Of course, these complications may be increased by the relative and subjective definitions of each student, teacher, administrator, and parent's view regarding if and how socioeconomic and social statuses are linked to bullying. There are many challenges associated with social, community, and individual inequalities that seriously limit the successful implementation and sustaining of policies to ameliorate violence and bullying within schools.

As discussed by previous researchers [41, 51], the experiences of student-athletes vary depending on how the particular school culture values students who participate in school sports. How student-athletes or school band members are perceived by other students differ from school to school, which could influence the relationship between social status and victimization. It is found that student-athletes are viewed as popular, central in social networks, and are extended preferential treatment in schools and communities that have high regard for interscholastic school sports; however, there are school cultures that promote the importance of academic success and honor societies where students with high grades and achievement scores are viewed as popular, central in social networks, and extended preferential treatment in schools and communities [11, 12]. Thus, school culture and the factors associated with the social status hierarchy could influence who is identified as popular or marginalized.

As highlighted in the introductory chapter, the concept of intersectionality also matters when understanding how socioeconomic and social statuses are associated with school bullying. For instance, students with lower socioeconomic status who attend disadvantaged schools and reside within a community that sustains high levels of disorder, and who are perceived as "weak" or "geeks" because of their academic success, are significantly more susceptible to victimization at school.

Conclusion

Although we attempt here to explicate socioeconomic and social statuses associated with school bullying, there is much more research needed to sufficiently understand and address bullying among disadvantaged and socially isolated or marginalized youth whose experiences are embedded in the complex group, school, community, and social and cultural contexts. While we have examined emerging literature highlighting some of the ways these contexts impact the school experiences of these disadvantaged and socially vulnerable student populations, we argue that additional research needs to investigate the risk and protective factors among these groups. Moreover, beyond additional efforts to identify these factors and their workings, we assert that the development of culturally appropriate intervention programs to strengthen and protect disadvantaged and socially vulnerable students in schools is paramount toward addressing school bullying victimization. Finally, we would like to remind the reader that factors raised in this chapter about socioeconomic and social statuses and school bullying victimization can also intersect with family cohesion and interaction, sex, sexual orientation, gender identity and expression, race, ethnicity, immigration, religion, disabilities, and special health needs.

References

1. Kozol, J. (2012). *Savage inequalities: Children in America's schools*. Broadway Books.
2. Lareau, A. (2011). *Unequal childhoods: Class, race, and family life*. University of California Press.
3. Lewis, A. E., & Diamond, J. B. (2017). *Despite the best intentions: How racial inequality thrives in good schools*. Oxford University Press.
4. Shedd, C. (2015). *Unequal city: Race, schools, and perceptions of injustice*. Russell Sage Foundation.
5. Hong, J. S. (2009). Feasibility of the Olweus bullying prevention program in low-income schools. *Journal of School Violence, 8*(1), 81–97.
6. Brunson, R. K., & Miller, J. (2009). Schools, neighborhoods, and adolescent conflicts: A situational examination of reciprocal dynamics. *Justice Quarterly, 26*(2), 183–210.
7. Sykes, B. L., Piquero, A. R., & Gioviano, J. P. (2017). Code of the classroom? Social disadvantage and bullying among American adolescents, US 2011-2012. *Crime & Delinquency, 63*(14), 1883–1922.
8. Suitts, S. (2015). *A new majority research bulletin: Low income students now a majority in the nation's public schools*. Southern Education Foundation.
9. Coleman, J. S. (1961). *The adolescent society: The social life of the teenager and its Impact on Education*. Glencoe, IL: Free Press.
10. Faris, R. (2012). Aggression, exclusivity, and status attainment in interpersonal networks. *Social Forces, 90*(4), 1207–1235.
11. Faris, R., & Felmlee, D. (2011). Status struggles: Network centrality and gender segregation in same-and cross-gender aggression. *American Sociological Review, 76*(1), 48–73.
12. Faris, R., & Felmlee, D. (2014). Casualties of social combat: School networks of peer victimization and their consequences. *American Sociological Review, 79*(2), 228–257.

13. Peguero, A. A. (2009). Opportunity, involvement, and student exposure to school violence. *Youth Violence and Juvenile Justice, 7*(4), 299–312.
14. Rodkin, P. C., & Berger, C. (2008). Who bullies whom? Social status asymmetries by victim gender. *International Journal of Behavioral Development, 32*(6), 473–485.
15. Salmivalli, C. (2010). Bullying and the peer group: A review. *Aggression and Violent Behavior, 15*(2), 112–120.
16. Juvonen, J., & Galvin, A. (n.d.). Peer influence in involuntary social groups: Lessons from research on bullying. In M. Prinstein & K. Dodge (Eds.), *Peer influence processes among youth* (pp. 225–244). New York: Guilford Press.
17. Espelage, D. L., Green, H. D., Jr., & Wasserman, S. (2007). Statistical analysis of friendship patterns and bullying behaviors among youth. *New Directions for Child and Adolescent Development, 2007*(118), 61–75.
18. Carolan, B. V. (2014). *Social network analysis and education: Theory, methods & applications*. Sage Publications.
19. Ahn, H.-J., & Rodkin, P. C. (2014). Classroom-level predictors of the social status of aggression: Friendship centralization, friendship density, teacher-student attunement, and gender. *Journal of Educational Psychology, 106*(4), 1144.
20. Twemlow, S. W., Fonagy, P., & Sacco, F. C. (2004). The role of the bystander in the social architecture of bullying and violence in schools and communities. *Annals of the New York Academy of Sciences, 1036*, 215–232.
21. Saarento, S., & Salmivalli, C. (2015). The role of classroom peer ecology and bystanders' responses in bullying. *Child Development Perspectives, 9*(4), 201–205.
22. Polanin, J. R., Espelage, D. L., & Pigott, T. D. (2012). A meta-analysis of school-based bullying prevention programs' effects on bystander intervention behavior. *School Psychology Review, 41*(1), 47–65.
23. Twemlow, S. W., & Sacco, F. C. (2013). How & why does bystanding have such a startling impact on the architecture of school bullying and violence? *International Journal of Applied Psychoanalytic Studies, 10*(3), 289–306.
24. Massey, D. S. (2007). *Categorically unequal: The American stratification system*. Russell Sage Foundation.
25. Roscigno, V. J., Tomaskovic-Devey, D., & Crowley, M. (2006). Education and the inequalities of place. *Social Forces, 84*(4), 2121–2145.
26. Ttofi, M. M., & Farrington, D. P. (2011). Effectiveness of school-based programs to reduce bullying: A systematic and meta-analytic review. *Journal of Experimental Criminology, 7*(1), 27–56.
27. Peguero, A. A., Popp, A. M., Latimore, T. L., Shekarkhar, Z., & Koo, D. J. (2011). Social control theory and school misbehavior: Examining the role of race and ethnicity. *Youth Violence and Juvenile Justice, 9*(3), 259–275.
28. Ansary, N. S., Elias, M. J., Greene, M. B., & Green, S. (2015). Guidance for schools selecting antibullying approaches: Translating evidence-based strategies to contemporary implementation realities. *Educational Researcher, 44*(1), 27–36.
29. Durán, R. (2012). *Gang life in two cities: An insider's journey*. Columbia University Press.
30. Finkelhor, D. (2014). *Childhood victimization: Violence, crime, and abuse in the lives of young people*. New York: Oxford University Press.
31. Bradshaw, C. P. (2017). *Handbook on bullying prevention: A life course perspective*. NASW Press.
32. Gottfredson, D. C. (2001). *Schools and delinquency*. New York: Cambridge University Press.
33. Addington, L. A., & Yablon, Y. B. (2011). How safe do students feel at school and while traveling to school? A comparative look at Israel and the United States. *American Journal of Education, 117*, 465–493.
34. Hughes, M. R., Gaines, J. S., & Pryor, D. W. (2015). Staying away from school: Adolescents who miss school due to feeling unsafe. *Youth Violence and Juvenile Justice, 13*, 270–290.

35. Varjas, K., Henrich, C. C., & Meyers, J. (2009). Urban middle school student's perceptions of bullying, cyberbullying, and school safety. *Journal of School Violence, 8*, 159–176.
36. Gottfredson, D. C., & DiPietro, S. M. (2011). School size, social capital, and student victimization. *Sociology of Education, 84*(1), 69–89.
37. Gottfredson, D. C. (2017). Prevention research in schools: Past, present, and future. *Criminology & Public Policy, 16*(1), 7–27.
38. Hutzell, K. L., & Payne, A. A. (2012). The impact of bullying victimization on school avoidance. *Youth Violence and Juvenile Justice, 10*(4), 370–385.
39. Hirschi, T. (1969). *Causes of delinquency*. Berkeley: University of California Press.
40. Payne, A. A., Gottfredson, D. C., & Gottfredson, G. D. (2003). Schools as communities: The relationships among communal school organization, student bonding, and school disorder. *Criminology, 41*(3), 749–778.
41. Peguero, A. A. (2008). Bullying victimization and extracurricular activity. *Journal of School Violence, 7*(3), 71–85.
42. Hindelang, M. J., Gottfredson, M. R., & Garofalo, J. (1978). *Victims of personal crime: An empirical foundation for a theory of personal victimization*. Cambridge, MA: Ballinger.
43. Popp, A. M. (2012). The difficulty in measuring suitable targets when modeling victimization. *Violence and Victims, 27*(5), 689–709.
44. Popp, A. M. (2012). The effects of exposure, proximity, and capable guardians on the risk of bullying victimization. *Youth Violence and Juvenile Justice, 10*(4), 315–332.
45. Wilcox, P., Tillyer, M. S., & Fisher, B. S. (2009). Gendered opportunity? School-based adolescent victimization. *Journal of Research in Crime and Delinquency, 46*(2), 245–269.
46. Kupchik, A. (2010). *Homeroom security: School discipline in an age of fear* (Vol. 6). NYU Press.
47. Kupchik, A. (2016). *The real school safety problem: The long-term consequences of harsh school punishment*. University of California Press.
48. Rios, V. M. (2011). *Punished: Policing the lives of Black and Latino boys*. NYU Press.
49. Rios, V. M. (2017). *Human targets: Schools, police, and the criminalization of Latino youth*. University of Chicago Press.
50. Peguero, A. A. (2012). Schools, bullying, and inequality: Intersecting factors and complexities with the stratification of youth victimization at school. *Sociology Compass, 6*(5), 402–412.
51. Kreager, D. A. (2007). Unnecessary roughness? School sports, peer networks, and male adolescent violence. *American Sociological Review, 72*(5), 705–724.

Chapter 4
The Role of the Family: Parents/Guardians, Siblings, Cohesion, and Interactions

Abstract In this chapter, we demonstrate how the role of the family, specifically parents/guardians, siblings, cohesion, and interactions affect the likelihood of being bullied. Several aspects of the home environment may be particularly relevant for victims of school bullying, as they may promote resilience in children going through this stressful experience. We also denote how bullied youth who have strong and intimate bonds or relationships with their parents/guardians might have more favorable psychosocial outcomes than would otherwise be the case. We present how youth from families with a culture of violence or maltreatment may feel powerless, as they are unable to protect themselves from harm and bullies. These youth are also likely to develop poor social skills, making them targets of bullying victimization and social exclusion.

Keywords Family cohesion · Family conflict · Parents/guardians · Siblings

Introduction

In this chapter, we examine the relevance of parents, guardians, siblings, and family cohesion and interactions in adolescents' school bullying involvement. Although adolescence is a period during which youth rely less on family members and more on friends and peers for social support, developmental psychologists contend that an individual's first socialization occurs in the home, and how they relate with their family can shape their relationships and socialization with their peers and others outside the home. The family has been defined as a system which comprises connected components (i.e., family members) that are organized around various functions that interact to maintain a balance and a state of equilibrium [1, p. 70]. Within the past several decades, the American family structure has undergone major changes [2], with an increasing number of immigrants, same-sex parents, single-parent, and blended family households.

We first discuss the family context in adolescents' bullying involvement from a social-ecological perspective, which is then followed by an adolescent's relations with their parents and guardian, and how that can foster or inhibit the risk

A. A. Peguero, J. S. Hong, *School Bullying*, Springer Series on Child and Family Studies, https://doi.org/10.1007/978-3-030-64367-6_4

of bullying and peer victimization in school. Next, we describe the role of sibling and sibling bullying, and how they can predispose or mitigate adolescents' bullying risks. We then discuss the role of family cohesion and interactions and how they are relevant to adolescents' bullying involvement. And finally, we discuss the family context of adolescent bullying within a social-ecological framework.

Overview of Adolescent Bullying Involvement Linked to Family Factors

Numerous studies have documented a link between parental factors and youths' involvement in bullying. Studies consistently show that parents of bullies and victims have been characterized as being punitive, displaying abusive and neglectful behavior, not showing warmth, and lacking monitoring. However, research to date has not examined the prevalence of parents or caregivers of youths identified as bullies and victims. For cyberbullying, one study [3] reported that compared to uninvolved students, cyberbullies and cyberbully/victims reported having poorer emotional bonds with their parents and lower levels of parental monitoring. About 30% of parents of cyberbullies and cyberbullying victims reported restricting their children's Internet use, which negatively affected children's willingness to disclose bullying incidents to parents [3]. One study [4] in the Netherlands also found that more than half of parents set rules about their children's Internet use, and in 8 out of 10 cases, they reported that they had rules about what was permitted activities on the Internet. However, parents' views about children's involvement in cyberbullying were also found to be contrary to what children had reported [see 5].

It is also challenging to estimate the prevalence rates of sibling bullying, considering that within the home, sibling competition, and conflict, which can manifest as sibling bullying, are quite frequent. A recent review of the literature suggests that while siblings experience some conflicts occasionally, up to 40% report experiencing sibling bullying every week [6]. It is important to note, however, that the prevalence rates appear to differ according to the type of aggression. One study [7] found that 32% of adolescents had reported experiencing a significantly higher rate of physical victimization by a sibling within the last year (32%) than property-based (10%) or psychological victimization (3%) [7].

Parents/guardians, siblings, and family members play a pivotal role in adolescents' socialization. Given that home is the first environmental context in which the developing child's socialization occurs, it is safe to assert that an adolescent's relations and interactions in the home can help predict the quality of his or her relationships with peers.

Parents/Guardians

Parents play a critical role in the development of their children's cognitive, social, and emotional health; and attachment, social support, and family systems are widely recognized theoretical conceptualizations of the relationship between the parent and the child [8]. Most parents would never purposely condone bullying or encourage their child to be involved in bullying behavior. However, parents can influence adolescents' bullying involvement, as they are significant contributors to the development of their children's relations with their peers, both directly (e.g., being involved in children's peer relationship skills) and indirectly (e.g., parental attitudes; [9]). Research has found that bullying involvement of adolescents is related to certain parental characteristics, such as parental support and protection, parental attitudes [10], parental relationship and conflict [3, 11], and parental discipline and maltreatment [12–14]. Studies also suggest that parents of bullies are hostile, rejecting, and indifferent to their children [13, 15], controlling [16], and usually inconsistent in a discipline [17]. In terms of parenting style, several studies also reported that parents of adolescents identified as bullies and victims tended to be authoritarian [18–20] among the four dimensions of parenting practices identified by Steinberg and his colleagues [21, 22]—*authoritative*, *authoritarian*, *indulgent*, and *neglectful.* Stevens, Bourdeaudhuij, and Oost [23] explored the differences between families of bullies, victims, bully/victims, and noninvolved children on family functioning, and parenting practices. Youth identified as bullies described their family as less cohesive, more conflictual, and less organized and controlled. Like bullies, youth identified as bullying victims reported more parental conflicts and punishments, and less close parent-youth relations.

Also, numerous studies have demonstrated unequivocally the importance of parental awareness and involvement in children's schooling for maximizing their academic potential. Studies have recognized the importance of parental awareness and involvement in children's bullying situation. In a sample of 251 child-parent pairs, Shemesh and colleagues [24] found that parents were aware of child-reported bullying in 52.1% of the cases, and parental awareness of bullying was found to be associated with a better quality of life and less distress in bullied children. In terms of perceptions, however, studies also report major differences in parents' reports versus children's reports of bullying. From a sample of 205 fifth grade students and their parents, Holt and colleagues' [9] findings suggest that children reported higher rates of bullying perpetration and victimization than parents, and parents were unaware of their children bullying others. Similarly, Stockdale, Hangaduambo, Duys, Larson, and Sarvela [25] also found from a sample of 739 fourth, fifth, and sixth graders, 367 parents, and 37 teachers in seven rural elementary schools that students tended to report a higher prevalence of bullying than did parents. Interestingly, one study [26] which collected data at three different time points, found that students tend to report lower overall peer victimization than did their parents and lower level of verbal victimization than did their teachers.

As for parents who are aware of their child being bullied in school, it is not uncommon for them to feel powerless and frustrated when they hear about their children's bullying situations. Empirical studies have documented a serious lack of contact between schools and parents in children's bullying situations. A review of research on parents' perspectives on children's bullying involvement by Harcourt, Jasperse, and Green [27] has documented that teachers and school officials rarely inform parents about the child's bullying situation, even when parents had to raise the concerns themselves [28], and parents often learn about their child's experience of bullying in other ways (e.g., child informing parents, parents guessing after a change in their child's behavior; [29]). Moreover, several cases of parents taking matters into their own hands in handling their child's bullying situations have been featured in news headlines. One case involved a Florida mother who strangled a 14-year-old boy who had tormented her 14-year-old daughter via Facebook. Another case involved a 53-year-old father in Brisbane, Australia, who strangled his teenage daughter's tormentor.

Despite the lack of direct connection between parents and schools, parents have been implicated in several bullying prevention efforts, particularly those involving parent–teacher collaborations and parental support [30, 31]. Parental support appears to buffer the effects of bullying on adverse psychosocial outcomes [30–32]. Conners-Burrow and colleagues' [31] study, which investigated the degree to which support from parents and teachers might moderate depressive symptoms in 977 fifth, ninth, and 11th-grade children who are victims, bullies, bully-victims, or uninvolved, reported that these children reported fewer symptoms of depression when parental support was high. The study also found that when parental support was high, the impact of teacher support was not significant. However, there are several challenges in parental support and involvement in bullying prevention efforts in school, including discrepancies in children's reporting of their experiences in peer victimization and parents' awareness of their children's experiences [33]. Another challenge is the difference between parental expectations and school officials' response when parents report their child's bullying incidents to the school officials [34].

Siblings

Case 1 *A twelve-year-old boy roughhouses with his eight-year-old brother and always wins. The older boy makes a point to rub it in. The eight-year-old complains that he has stomachaches and headaches when he comes home from school. He complains to his parents who are both at work and his father tells him that he "need[s] to 'man up' and fight back if [you're] going to make it in the real world. The eight-year-old boy gets sadder and withdrawn while his older brother gets more brazen with his taunting"* [35].

Case 2 *Tanya, eleven, sat in her room crying. Her right cheek is still red from the slap she received from her sister, Carissa. Carissa is thirteen-years-old and has been abusing Tanya for weeks. Last week, she received a bruise on her leg after her sister kicked her. Tanya doesn't understand why her sister despised her. She loves her older sister but felt her sister thought she was her parents' favorite. The words Carissa called her repeatedly echoed over and over again in her head. "Ugly," "Stupid," "Bitch." When Tanya told others about all this, she was told that it's not unusual for sisters to not get along and fighting is always normal* [36].

Although most individuals in the U.S. grow up with at least one sibling, and although sibling relationships are often the longest-lasting relationships in an individual's life, research on sibling relationships is limited in comparison to that on other relationships in the family [37]. Although recent evidence suggests that bullying among siblings, or sibling bullying, can be carried out repeatedly and is frequent, few studies have explored bullying and aggression involving siblings. A high prevalence of sibling bullying has been reported in several of these studies. Skinner and Kowalski [38] found from a sample of 27 sibling pairs that 78% reported being victimized by their sibling and 85% reported bullying their sibling during childhood. A longitudinal study conducted by Tippett and Wolke [39] also found that sibling bullying was widespread, with 46% of all study participants being victimized and 36% perpetrating bullying toward their peers. A review of research on sibling bullying also reported that sibling bullying is frequent with up to 50% involved in bullying every month [40]. Several studies also reported a higher frequency of sibling bullying than peer bullying among adolescents. One study, which compared 392 young adults' experiences with a sibling and peers bullying during childhood, found that although the participants viewed peer bullying and sibling bullying as similar, sibling bullying behavior was reported to be perpetrated and experienced more often [41]. Another study, which consisted of 455 children in grades 5–12, showed that the percentage of sibling bullying perpetration was significantly higher than peer bullying perpetration (31.6% vs. 9.8%) [42].

According to Malecki and Demaray [43], five signs that indicate that sibling fighting may be bullying are: (1) fighting among siblings seems more intense than expected, (2) there are patterns to the fighting, (3) during the altercations, one sibling appears consistently to be more powerful than the other, (4) the siblings don't "make up" after a fight, and (5) the perpetrator shows a lack of empathy. Also, risk factors for sibling bullying, particularly at the individual and relational levels have been documented in the empirical literature. Boys are more often victims [44], perpetrators, or bully/victims, whereas girls are more often victims of sibling bullying [45]. The presence of an older brother, anger trait, moral disengagement, low level of empathy, low socio-economic status, family disorganization, parental violence, and peer bullying at school were also found to be associated with sibling bullying in other studies [39, 42, 45–47].

Sibling bullying can harm children's mental health and psychosocial development [6, 7, 48, 49]. In a study involving a national probability sample that included telephone interviews, Tucker and colleagues [7] found that children ages 0–9 and youth ages 10–17 who experienced sibling aggression in the past year reported greater mental health distress. From a community-based birth cohort study in the United Kingdom, Bowes and colleagues [48] also found that children who were frequently bullied by their sibling were twice as likely to have depression, engage in self-harm, and display anxiety compared to children who were not bullied by their sibling. Exposure to sibling violence (perpetration and victimization) is a risk factor for not only impaired psychological functioning (internalizing and externalizing problems) but also for impaired academic competence [50], and risk behaviors such as substance use, aggression, and delinquency [51]. From a study using data from the 2007 Secondary School Student Survey ($N = 8122$), Button and Gealt [51] also reported that sibling violence occurs more frequently than other forms of abuse. Likewise there, sibling violence was also found to be significantly related to substance use, aggression, and delinquency [51].

Family Conflict, Family Cohesion, and Adolescent Bullying

The family systems framework may provide an important perspective on family antecedents of bullying and peer victimization. *Family functioning* is conceptualized as a process that involves "the integration and maintenance of the family unit and its ability to carry out essential tasks for the growth and well-being of its members, such as the nurturance and protection of offspring...." [52]. Two major aspects of family functioning that empirically support their link with bullying include family conflict and family cohesion [53]. *Family conflict* is defined as openly expressed anger, aggression, and conflict among members of the family [54], which can also include covert/overt forms of fighting, arguing, blaming acceptance of personal responsibility, and negative feelings in the family [55]. *Family cohesion* is characterized as emotional bonding and feeling of closeness among family members, which can be expressed by feelings of acceptance and belonging [56]. In the 1930s, sociologist Angell [57] identified cohesion as an important aspect of interactions among family members, and in the late 1970s, Olson, Sprenkle, and Russell [58] identified two important components of family cohesion: "the emotional bonding members have with one another and the degree of individual autonomy a person experiences in the family system" [p. 5]. Family cohesion has been implicated in research on children's and adolescents' psychosocial development, including internalizing problems, academic achievement, and risk behaviors [59–62]. Not surprisingly, families characterized as displaying high levels of cohesion (i.e., warmth, and lower levels of hostility) have been found to have optimal family functioning and be less likely to have a child who is involved in bullying. Empirical evidence on the relationship between family cohesion and bullying have compared bullies, victims, bully/victims, or uninvolved on their mean differences in family cohesion. Extant studies have consistently found that youth identified as bullies display a lower level of family cohesion than their victimized or uninvolved peers [23, 63, 64]. These studies consistently show that positive family characteristics such as family cohesion can reduce adolescents' tendency to be involved in peer conflicts and bullying.

Social-Ecological Framework

As Bronfenbrenner had postulated, a *family* is a principal context in which an individual's developmental process and behavior take place [65]. Although bullying occurs most frequently in the school setting where adolescents have frequent interactions with peer groups, the processes operating in the one setting (e.g., school) can be impacted by those in another setting (e.g., home) [65]. In other words, adolescent bullying involvement does not occur in isolation and does not exclusively occur in one context. Bullying is a phenomenon characterized as a complex social exchange among individuals, groups, and the social environment. In this chapter, the social-ecological framework is divided into four-level factors: societal, community, (peer) group, and individual.

Societal

The societal level highlights cultural, institutional, and structural factors, and how the link between adolescents' involvement in bullying and family relations can be shaped by such societal level factors as broad sets of cultural values and beliefs, which permeate and influence the family microsystems. *Culture* is conceived of as a set of distinctive patterns of beliefs and behaviors that are influenced by a group of people, which serve to regulate their daily living [66]. Culture has been a viable tool for constructing parenting practices. In the U.S., there has been a growing trend toward society becoming more ethnically and culturally diverse, which has also transformed parenting practices. Research investigating cultural values and parenting, and how this link is associated with adolescents' bullying is sparse, although parents are widely perceived as having the utmost responsibility for socializing their children [67]. In general, there have not been any studies exploring how societal factors can shape relations and interactions in the family which in turn might contribute to adolescents' problem behaviors, such as bullying involvement. However, studies have found, for example, that beliefs supportive of violence and masculine norms can influence both parenting practices and adolescent bullying behavior [68, 69]. Considering that children have traditionally had lower status in society and within the family than adults, and physical punishment is regarded as an acceptable part of child-rearing practice [70], it is not surprising that there is strong evidence of an association between societal norms supportive of violence and parental abuse [e.g., see 70], which, in turn, can contribute to children's aggressive behaviors outside the home.

Community

Community contexts in which interpersonal relationships occur such as home and the school can also influence adolescents' behavior and their risk of problematic peer relationships (e.g., bullying involvement). Also, several neighborhood and community influences are significant when considering parenting behaviors and youth outcomes; home and school are embedded in the community, and extant research has demonstrated a strong link between community-level factors (e.g., crime and violence in the community) and parenting practices. Several study findings suggest a positive link between community violence and parental abuse at home, as it has long been recognized that poverty is highly correlated with child maltreatment [71]. Economic hardships in the community and income loss in families in the city of Oakland during the Great Depression in the 1930s were reportedly concurrent with a decrease in parental nurturance, and an increase in inconsistent and punitive parenting practices [72, 73]. The effectiveness of parenting practices can also vary by neighborhood conditions and community contexts [74]. Researchers [e.g., 75] also observed how community violence and maltreatment in the home interact in producing adverse consequences for children and adolescents' development and socialization [p. 98; also see 74]. The detrimental effects of exposure to violence in the community are present in some adolescents residing in a high-risk community. More specifically, feelings of insecurity and alterations in social cognition from exposure to violence in the community and the home can potentially affect children's relationships with their peers, as numerous studies have found evidence of problematic peer relations such as bullying and aggressive behaviors [76] among children who have been exposed to violence [see 76, for a review].

During the past decade, several researchers have also focused on community social organization and collective efficacy, including social capital, formal and informal networks, and community capacity building (i.e., the degree to which residents in the community demonstrate a sense of shared responsibility for the welfare of the residents, as well as demonstrate collective competence by utilizing opportunities for addressing community needs and confront situations that may threaten the safety and well-being of the residents; [74]). Such social ties and interactions in the communities can positively address problems, such as problem behavior of adolescents. One study also found that collective efficacy in the community was negatively associated with problem behaviors of adolescents related to permissive parenting [74, 77]: high levels of collective efficacy can increase the quality of parenting, as adults in the community can put pressure on the parents and caretakers of misbehaving adolescents to become more responsible caretakers [74, 78].

Group

It is often stated that bullying is a group process [79]. Developmental psychologists have long argued that individuals rely less on their parents and more on their peer groups as a source of socialization and social support [80]. Indeed, peer group relations are a central component of adolescent development. However, the family remains an important context, which can shape an individual's relations and interactions within a peer group [81]. There is empirical support for Bronfenbrenner's [82] mesosystem influence on adolescent development, specifically, how proximal processes in one microsystem (family) may influence an individual's relationships in another (peer group) [83]. The quality of the relationships within peer groups can also be shaped by an adolescent's perceptions of his or her parental relations [see 83], as well as their perceptions of parenting style. For instance, authoritative parenting can encourage adolescents to be less susceptible to peer group influence in domains in which peer groups engage in negative behaviors [84], such as being involved in bullying. On the other hand, negative behavior toward peers and peer groups has been seen as emanating from a failure in bonding with a parent figure. For example, an earlier study [85] has found that highly dominating parents are more likely than others to have children who have negative relations with their peer groups because they are replicating behaviors that are modeled for them in the home [86]. However, it is also important to remember that although family and peer groups can exert negative influences on adolescents, they can also exert positive influences. A study by Rigby and Johnson [87] found that youth who reported that their friends and parents expected them to support victimized adolescents were not only less likely to be involved in bullying but were also more likely to intervene in bullying incidents.

Individual

An understanding of the importance of considering the individual within the context of the family as old as the field of psychiatry, which began with Sigmund Freud's preoccupation with the influence of the individual family on early childhood development and psychopathology [88]. More recently, the recognition of the importance of examining the individual in the context of the family dynamics and relationship patterns is reflected more broadly, in various fields and most notably, in the field of psychology [88]. Individual-level family characteristics, such as parent-child conflict, maltreatment, and family dissonance have been implicated in research on adolescents' involvement in bullying dynamics [e.g., 9, 88].

There is also a small but growing literature that suggests that certain family relations, behavior, and dynamics might protect individuals from bullying involvement, even among children who are otherwise in contexts that might put them at significant risk. Having supportive families can buffer youth involved in bullying from developing adjustment problems by providing social supports, reducing stress, or encouraging youth to develop coping mechanisms to deal with bullying [89]. Further, the link between family factors and youths' psychosocial adjustment following bullying involvement may be reflective of genetic influences. For instance, parents who provide a caring home environment and those who have positive parenting skills may also pass on to their children genes that are associated with resilience [89].

Complexities

Although the linkage between family-level factors—for example, parenting practices, sibling relations, and family conflicts—and adolescents' involvement in bullying has been supported empirically, there are also limitations to the extant studies. It is important to recognize the changing family structure in the U.S. over the past several decades, which includes growing rates of single-mother households, same-sex households, and non-family households. According to the U.S. Census Bureau, in the 1940s, married couples made up 76.5 percent of American households while single-parent and non-family households included 10 percent of all households [90]. In 2010, 48.4% of all households consisted of married couples while 33.6% included non-family arrangements [90]. However, there are very few studies that have explored the parenting practices of caregivers in "non-traditional" households and how that may be related to adolescents' involvement in bullying. It is important to recognize that although families may provide social and economic support to dependents (children), an individual's psychosocial well-being can be heavily influenced by parenting practices and by his or her living arrangements.

Moreover, although parenting practices and their association with adolescent bullying and peer relationships have been researched extensively, many studies have not explored racial and ethnic differences in parenting practices, and how they may influence or inhibit adolescents' bullying involvement. One of a few studies, Hong, Ryou, and Piquero [91] explored racial differences in parenting and how they may buffer against bullying perpetration and peer victimization. The study found that White/European American and Black/African Americans were both less likely to report being bullied if they received parental/guardian support and were satisfied with their family. Further, a mother's parental monitoring was also found to be negatively associated with bullying and peer victimization for both racial groups. However, a father's parental monitoring was only found to be negatively associated with bullying and peer victimization among White/European American adolescents only [91]. Future studies must consider racial and ethnic differences in parenting practices in adolescents' bullying involvement. A consideration of racial and ethnic differences is important, given that parents are frequently implicated in bullying prevention and intervention efforts, and scholars and interventionists have advocated for home-school collaborations, involving parents as well as teachers and school officials. To illustrate, while "harsh parenting" and physical discipline are positively associated with externalizing and antisocial behavior in White/European American youth, it is not associated with such behavior in African American youth.

Conclusion

In this chapter, we explored how family dynamics and relationships in the home are associated with bullying involvement. Research has made a tremendous stride in enhancing our understanding of this association. However, there is much more research needed to understand how family relations-peer relations might vary when we consider social identities, including race/ethnicity, health/mental health status, sexual orientation, socio-economic status, and so forth. Further, we have identified significant emerging literature that highlights some of how family-level risk factors such as maltreatment and parent/sibling conflicts may reinforce problematic peer relationships in adolescents. However, we also strongly argue that more in-depth research taking into consideration protective factors occurring in multiple systems levels, including societal, community, group, and individual, is needed. And finally, we would like to remind the readers that bullying and peer victimization are one of many by-products of the complex interplay between inter- and intra-individual variables [92].

References

1. McWhirter, J. J., McWhirter, B. T., McWhirter, E. H., & McWhirter, R. J. (2007). *At risk youth*. Belmont, CA: Thomson Brooks/Cole.
2. Halpern, D. F. (2005). Psychology at the intersection of work and family: Recommendations for employers, working families, and policymakers. *American Psychologist, 60*(5), 397.
3. Ybarra, M. L., & Mitchell, K. J. (2004). Youth engaging in online harassment: Associations with caregiver–child relationships, internet use, and personal characteristics. *Journal of Adolescence, 27*(3), 319–336.
4. Dehue, F., Bolman, C., & Völlink, T. (2008). Cyberbullying: Youngsters' experiences and parental perception. *Cyberpsychology & Behavior, 11*(2), 217–223.
5. Zych, I., Baldry, A. C., & Farrington, D. P. (2017). School bullying and cyberbullying: Prevalence, characteristics, outcomes, and prevention. In Handbook of behavioral criminology (pp. 113–138). Springer.
6. Wolke, D., Tippett, N., & Dantchev, S. (2015). Bullying in the family: Sibling bullying. *The Lancet Psychiatry, 2*(10), 917–929.
7. Tucker, C. J., Finkelhor, D., Shattuck, A. M., & Turner, H. (2013). Prevalence and correlates of sibling victimization types. *Child Abuse & Neglect, 37*(4), 213–223.
8. Nickerson, A. B., Mele, D., & Osborne-Oliver, K. (2010). Parent-child relationships and bullying. In S. R. Jimerson, S. M. Swearer, & D. L. Espelage (Eds.), *Handbook of bullying in school: An international perspective* (pp. 187–210). New York & Oxon: Routledge.
9. Holt, M. K., Kaufman Kantor, G., & Finkelhor, D. (2008). Parent/child concordance about bullying involvement and family characteristics related to bullying and peer victimization. *Journal of School Violence, 8*(1), 42–63.
10. Eslea, M., & Smith, P. K. (2000). Pupil and parent attitudes towards bullying in primary schools. *European Journal of Psychology of Education, 15*(2), 207–219.
11. Georgiou, S. N., & Stavrinides, P. (2013). Parenting at home and bullying at school. *Social Psychology of Education, 16*(2), 165–179.
12. Baldry, A. C., & Farrington, D. P. (2005). Protective factors as moderators of risk factors in adolescence bullying. *Social Psychology of Education, 8*(3), 263–284.
13. Kokkinos, C. M., & Panayiotou, G. (2007). Parental discipline practices and locus of control: Relationship to bullying and victimization experiences of elementary school students. *Social Psychology of Education, 10*(3), 281–301.
14. Shields, A., & Cicchetti, D. (2001). Parental maltreatment and emotion dysregulation as risk factors for bullying and victimization in middle childhood. *Journal of Clinical Child Psychology, 30*(3), 349–363.

15. Smokowski, P. R., & Kopasz, K. H. (2005). Bullying in school: An overview of types, effects, family characteristics, and intervention strategies. *Children & Schools, 27*(2), 101–110.
16. Curtner-Smith, M. E., Culp, A. M., Culp, R., Scheib, C., Owen, K., Tilley, A., et al. (2006). Mothers' parenting and young economically disadvantaged children's relational and overt bullying. *Journal of Child and Family Studies, 15*(2), 177–189.
17. Carney, A. G., & Merrell, K. W. (2001). Bullying in schools: Perspectives on understanding and preventing an international problem. *School Psychology International, 22*(3), 364–382.
18. Ahmed, E., & Braithwaite, V. (2004). Bullying and victimization: Cause for concern for both families and schools. *Social Psychology of Education, 7*(1), 35–54.
19. Baldry, A. C., & Farrington, D. P. (1998). Parenting influences on bullying and victimization. *Legal and Criminological Psychology, 3*(2), 237–254.
20. Georgiou, S. N., Fousiani, K., Michaelides, M., & Stavrinides, P. (2013). Cultural value orientation and authoritarian parenting as parameters of bullying and victimization at school. *International Journal of Psychology, 48*(1), 69–78.
21. Lamborn, S. D., Mounts, N. S., Steinberg, L., & Dornbusch, S. M. (1991). Patterns of competence and adjustment among adolescents from authoritative, authoritarian, indulgent, and neglectful families. *Child Development, 62*(5), 1049–1065.
22. Steinberg, L., Lamborn, S. D., Darling, N., Mounts, N. S., & Dornbusch, S. M. (1994). Over-time changes in adjustment and competence among adolescents from authoritative, authoritarian, indulgent, and neglectful families. *Child Development, 65*(3), 754–770.
23. Stevens, V., De Bourdeaudhuij, I., & Van Oost, P. (2002). Relationship of the family environment to children's involvement in bully/victim problems at school. *Journal of Youth and Adolescence, 31*(6), 419–428.
24. Shemesh, E., Annunziato, R. A., Ambrose, M. A., Ravid, N. L., Mullarkey, C., Rubes, M., et al. (2013). Child and parental reports of bullying in a consecutive sample of children with food allergy. *Pediatrics, 131*(1), e10–e17.
25. Stockdale, M. S., Hangaduambo, S., Duys, D., Larson, K., & Sarvela, P. D. (2002). Rural elementary students', parents', and teachers' perceptions of bullying. *American Journal of Health Behavior, 26*(4), 266–277.
26. Newgent, R. A., Lounsbery, K. L., Keller, E. A., Baker, C. R., Cavell, T. A., & Boughfman, E. M. (2009). Differential perceptions of bullying in the schools: A comparison of student, parent, teacher, school counselor, and principal reports. *Journal of School Counseling, 7*(38), n38.
27. Harcourt, S., Jasperse, M., & Green, V. A. (2014). "We were sad and we were angry": A systematic review of parents' perspectives on bullying. In Child & Youth Care Forum (Vol. 43, pp. 373–391). Springer.
28. Humphrey, G., & Crisp, B. R. (2008). Bullying affects us too: Parental responses to bullying at kindergarten. *Australasian Journal of Early Childhood, 33*(1), 45–49.
29. Brown, J. R. (2010). Trajectories of parents' experiences in discovering, reporting, and living with the aftermath of middle school bullying. Doctoral dissertation. Retrieved from ProQuest Dissertations and Theses (UMI No. 3409133).
30. Claes, L., Luyckx, K., Baetens, I., Van de Ven, M., & Witteman, C. (2015). Bullying and victimization, depressive mood, and non-suicidal self-injury in adolescents: The moderating role of parental support. *Journal of Child and Family Studies, 24*(11), 3363–3371.
31. Conners-Burrow, N. A., Johnson, D. L., Whiteside-Mansell, L., McKelvey, L., & Gargus, R. A. (2009). Adults matter: Protecting children from the negative impacts of bullying. *Psychology in the Schools, 46*(7), 593–604.
32. Antonio, R., & Moleiro, C. (2015). Social and parental support as moderators of the effects of homophobic bullying on psychological distress in youth. *Psychology in the Schools, 52*(8), 729–742.
33. Matsunaga, M. (2009). Parents don't (always) know their children have been bullied: Child-parent discrepancy on bullying and family-level profile of communication standards. *Human Communication Research, 35*(2), 221–247.

34. Brown, J. R., Aalsma, M. C., & Ott, M. A. (2013). The experiences of parents who report youth bullying victimization to school officials. *Journal of Interpersonal Violence, 28*(3), 494–518.
35. Krull, E. (2009). Bullying Between Siblings. Retrieved August 18, 2020, from https://blogs.psychcentral.com/family/2009/11/bullying-between-siblings/
36. Lohmann, R. C. (2014). Sibling bullying. *Psychology today*. Retrieved August 18, 2020, from http://www.psychologytoday.com/blog/teen-angst/201404/sibling-bullying
37. Whiteman, S. D., McHale, S. M., & Soli, A. (2011). Theoretical perspectives on sibling relationships. *Journal of Family Theory & Review, 3*(2), 124–139.
38. Skinner, J. A., & Kowalski, R. M. (2013). Profiles of sibling bullying. *Journal of Interpersonal Violence, 28*(8), 1726–1736.
39. Tippett, N., & Wolke, D. (2015). Aggression between siblings: Associations with the home environment and peer bullying. *Aggressive Behavior, 41*(1), 14–24.
40. Wolke, D., & Skew, A. J. (2012). Bullying among siblings. *International Journal of Adolescent Medicine and Health, 24*(1), 17–25.
41. Hoetger, L. A., Hazen, K. P., & Brank, E. M. (2015). All in the family: A retrospective study comparing sibling bullying and peer bullying. *Journal of Family Violence, 30*(1), 103–111.
42. Tanrikulu, I., & Campbell, M. A. (2015). Sibling bullying perpetration: Associations with gender, grade, peer perpetration, trait anger, and moral disengagement. *Journal of Interpersonal Violence, 30*(6), 1010–1024.
43. Malecki, C. K., & Demaray, M. K. (2014). 5 Signs that sibling fighting may be bullying. *Psychology today*. Retrieved August 18, 2020, from http://www.psychologytoday.com/blog/the-wide-wide-world-psychology/201412/5-signs-sibling-fighting-may-be-bullying
44. Duncan, R. D. (1999). Peer and sibling aggression: An investigation of intra-and extra-familial bullying. *Journal of Interpersonal Violence, 14*(8), 871–886.
45. Wolke, D., & Skew, A. J. (2011). Bullied at home and at school: Relationship to behavior problems and unhappiness. In S. McFall (Ed.), *Understanding society: Early findings from the first wave of the UK's household longitudinal study* (pp. 23–32). London: Economic Social Research Council.
46. Eriksen, S., & Jensen, V. (2006). All in the family? Family environment factors in sibling violence. *Journal of Family Violence, 21*(8), 497–507.
47. Menesini, E., Camodeca, M., & Nocentini, A. (2010). Bullying among siblings: The role of personality and relational variables. *British Journal of Developmental Psychology, 28*(4), 921–939.
48. Bowes, L., Wolke, D., Joinson, C., Lereya, S. T., & Lewis, G. (2014). Sibling bullying and risk of depression, anxiety, and self-harm: A prospective cohort study. *Pediatrics, 134*(4), e1032–e1039.
49. Fisher, H. L., Moffitt, T. E., Houts, R. M., Belsky, D. W., Arseneault, L., & Caspi, A. (2012). Bullying victimisation and risk of self harm in early adolescence: Longitudinal cohort study. *BMJ, 344*, 1–9.
50. Linares, L. O. (2006). An understudied form of intra-family violence: Sibling-to-sibling aggression among foster children. *Aggression and Violent Behavior, 11*(1), 95–109.
51. Button, D. M., & Gealt, R. (2010). High risk behaviors among victims of sibling violence. *Journal of Family Violence, 25*(2), 131–140.
52. Walsh, F. (Ed.). (1993). *Normal family processes*. New York: Guilford Press.
53. Sapp, R. L. (2003). *Family conflict and family cohesion: Their relationship to youths' behavior problems*. Knoxville: The University of Tennessee. Retrieved from https://trace.tennessee.edu/cgi/viewcontent.cgi?article=3729&context=utk_graddiss.
54. Moos, R. H., & Moos, B. S. (1994). *Family environment scale manual: Development, applications, research*. Palo Alto, CA: Consulting Psychologists Press.
55. Beavers, W. R., & Hampson, R. B. (1990). *Successful families: Assessment and intervention*. WW Norton.
56. McKeown, R. E., Garrison, C. Z., Jackson, K. L., Cuffe, S. P., Addy, C. L., & Waller, J. L. (1997). Family structure and cohesion, and depressive symptoms in adolescents. *Journal of Research on Adolescence, 7*(3), 267–281.

57. Angell, R. (1936). *The family encounters the depression. Scribner*. Simon & Schuster.
58. Olson, D. H., Sprenkle, D. H., & Russell, C. S. (1979). Circumplex model of marital and family systems: I. cohesion and adaptability dimensions, family types, and clinical applications. *Family Process, 18*(1), 3–28.
59. Annunziata, D., Hogue, A., Faw, L., & Liddle, H. A. (2006). Family functioning and school success in at-risk, inner-city adolescents. *Journal of Youth and Adolescence, 35*(1), 100–108.
60. Harris, T. L., & Molock, S. D. (2000). Cultural orientation, family cohesion, and family support in suicide ideation and depression among African American college students. *Suicide and Life-threatening Behavior, 30*(4), 341–353.
61. Johnson, H. D., Lavoie, J. C., & Mahoney, M. (2001). Interparental conflict and family cohesion: Predictors of loneliness, social anxiety, and social avoidance in late adolescence. *Journal of Adolescent Research, 16*(3), 304–318.
62. Marsiglia, F. F., Parsai, M., & Kulis, S. (2009). Effects of familism and family cohesion on problem behaviors among adolescents in Mexican immigrant families in the Southwest United States. *Journal of Ethnic & Cultural Diversity in Social Work, 18*(3), 203–220.
63. Berdondini, L., & Smith, P. K. (1996). Cohesion and power in the families of children involved in bully/victim problems at school: An Italian replication. *Journal of Family Therapy, 18*(1), 99–102.
64. van Hoof, A., Raaijmakers, Q. A., van Beek, Y., Hale, W. W., & Aleva, L. (2008). A multi-mediation model on the relations of bullying, victimization, identity, and family with adolescent depressive symptoms. *Journal of Youth and Adolescence, 37*(7), 772–782.
65. Bronfenbrenner, U. (1986). Ecology of the family as a context for human development: Research perspectives. *Developmental Psychology, 22*(6), 723.
66. Bornstein, M. H. (2012). Cultural approaches to parenting. *Parenting, 12*(2–3), 212–221.
67. Baumrind, D. (1978). Parental disciplinary patterns and social competence in children. *Youth & Society, 9*(3), 239–267.
68. Bosworth, K., Espelage, D. L., & Simon, T. R. (1999). Factors associated with bullying behavior in middle school students. *The Journal of Early Adolescence, 19*(3), 341–362.
69. Poteat, V. P., Kimmel, M. S., & Wilchins, R. (2011). The moderating effects of support for violence beliefs on masculine norms, aggression, and homophobic behavior during adolescence. *Journal of Research on Adolescence, 21*(2), 434–447.
70. World Health Organization. (2009). *Violence prevention: The evidence. Changing cultural and social norms that support violence*. Malta: World Health Organization.
71. Cicchetti, D., & Lynch, M. (1993). Toward an ecological/transactional model of community violence and child maltreatment: Consequences for children's development. *Psychiatry, 56*(1), 96–118.
72. Elder, G. H., Jr. (1974). *Children of the great depression*. Chicago, IL: University of Chicago Press.
73. Taylor, J., Spencer, N., & Baldwin, N. (2000). Social, economic, and political context of parenting. *Archives of Disease in Childhood, 82*(2), 113–120.
74. Hoskins, D. H. (2014). Consequences of parenting on adolescent outcomes. *Societies, 4*(3), 506–531.
75. Belsky, J. (1993). Etiology of child maltreatment: A developmental-ecological analysis. *Psychological Bulletin, 114*(3), 413.
76. Schwartz, D., & Proctor, L. J. (2000). Community violence exposure and children's social adjustment in the school peer group: The mediating roles of emotion regulation and social cognition. *Journal of Consulting and Clinical Psychology, 68*(4), 670.
77. Browning, C. R., Leventhal, T., & Brooks-Gunn, J. (2005). Sexual initiation in early adolescence: The nexus of parental and community control. *American Sociological Review, 70*(5), 758–778.
78. Simons, R. L., Simons, L. G., Burt, C. H., Brody, G. H., & Cutrona, C. (2005). Collective efficacy, authoritative parenting and delinquency: A longitudinal test of a model integrating community-and family-level processes. *Criminology, 43*(4), 989–1029.

79. Salmivalli, C. (2010). Bullying and the peer group: A review. *Aggression and Violent Behavior, 15*(2), 112–120.
80. Steinberg, L. (1993). *Adolescence*. McGraw-Hill.
81. Parke, R. D., & Bhavnagri, N. P. (1989). Parents as managers of children's peer relationships. In D. Belle (Ed.), *Children's social network and social support* (pp. 241–259). New York: Wiley.
82. Bronfenbrenner, U. (1977). Toward an experimental ecology of human development. *American Psychologist, 32*(7), 513.
83. Bogenschneider, K., Wu, M., Raffaelli, M., & Tsay, J. C. (1998). Parent influences on adolescent peer orientation and substance use: The interface of parenting practices and values. *Child Development, 69*(6), 1672–1688.
84. Mounts, N. S., & Steinberg, L. (1995). An ecological analysis of peer influence on adolescent grade point average and drug use. *Developmental Psychology, 31*(6), 915.
85. Manning, M., Heron, J., & Marshall, T. (1978). Styles of hostility and social interactions at nursery, at school and at home: An extended study of children. In *Aggression and anti-social behaviour in childhood and adolescence* (pp. 29–58). Oxford: Pergamon Press.
86. Bandura, A. (1977). Self-efficacy: Toward a unifying theory of behavioral change. *Psychological Review, 84*(2), 191.
87. Rigby, K., & Johnson, B. (2006). Expressed readiness of Australian schoolchildren to act as bystanders in support of children who are being bullied. *Educational Psychology, 26*(3), 425–440.
88. Szapocznik, J., & Kurtines, W. M. (1993). Family psychology and cultural diversity: Opportunities for theory, research, and application. *American Psychologist, 48*(4), 400.
89. Bowes, L., Maughan, B., Caspi, A., Moffitt, T. E., & Arseneault, L. (2010). Families promote emotional and behavioural resilience to bullying: Evidence of an environmental effect. *Journal of Child Psychology and Psychiatry, 51*(7), 809–817.
90. Population Reference Bureau (2012). Household Change in the United States – Population Reference Bureau. Retrieved from https://www.prb.org/us-household-change/
91. Hong, J. S., Ryou, B., & Piquero, A. R. (2018). Do family-level factors associated with bullying perpetration and peer victimization differ by race? Comparing European American and African American youth. *Journal of Interpersonal Violence*. https://doi.org/10.1177/0886260517714441.
92. Swearer, S. M., & Doll, B. (2001). Bullying in schools: An ecological framework. *Journal of Emotional Abuse, 2*(2–3), 7–23.

Chapter 5
Sex, Sexual Orientation, Gender Identity, and Gender Expression: Definitions and Implications for Marginalization

Abstract In this chapter, we examine how sex, sexual orientation, gender identity, and gender expression are linked to the likelihood of being bullied. We will also be defining the terms sex, sexual orientation, gender identity, and gender expression for our readers, especially in regards to school bullying. Next, we provide the patterns and disparities associated with each of these aforementioned classifications. Of course, we will present how sex, sexual orientation, gender identity, and gender expression with school bullying should be considered through a social-ecological framework.

Keywords Sex · Sexual orientation · Gender identity · Gender expression

Introduction

In this chapter, we focus on sex, sexual orientation, gender identity, and gender expression and how they are related to bullying. A great deal of research has focused on sex differences in bullying as well as homophobic bullying which is often motivated by actual or perceived minority sexual orientation, gender identity, and gender expression. Many studies have reported that in terms of sex differences, boys are more likely than girls to be involved in bullying. Concerning sexual orientation, gender identity, and gender expression, studies have found that youth identified as lesbian, gay, bisexual, transgender, and sexually questioning are significantly at risk of bullying victimization in school [1, 2]. Also, the emerging body of the research literature has found gender identity and (non-conforming) gender expression to be significant risk factors for bullying involvement—as a perpetrator, victim, or both.

Sex Differences

Biological sex is one of the strongest correlates of school bullying [3]. Not surprisingly, past studies have found that boys are more likely than girls to be involved in bullying, as males are considered the more "aggressive sex" [4]. Several empirical

A. A. Peguero, J. S. Hong, *School Bullying*, Springer Series on Child and Family Studies, https://doi.org/10.1007/978-3-030-64367-6_5

findings have documented that boys engaged in and were targets of face-to-face bullying more than girls [5–8]. Several studies have also reported significant differences in how boys bully versus how girls bully others [3; see 9 for a review]. Boys tend to be physically aggressive when bullying others and are likely to engage in direct forms of bullying—both physical (e.g., hitting, kicking, shoving) and verbal (e.g., calling names, taunting, and threatening). Girls, on the other hand, are more likely to engage in indirect forms of bullying through the peer group (e.g., gossiping, spreading rumors, excluding a target from their social group; [10]). Because girls use an indirect method of bullying, it can be difficult to recognize and detect. Girls may use their popularity status to discourage others from becoming friends with the victim. Many studies also report that girls are more frequently than boys to be engaged in a phenomenon known as "relational aggression," in which the goal is to harm others through purposeful manipulation and damaging the victim's relationships [4].

Several recent studies, however, found no gender differences in bullying, and a limited number of studies also reported that girls are more likely to be victimized than boys. According to the Ophelia Project, which collected data from 1882 students from 16 U.S. public and private schools (with an equal proportion of male and female students), girls reported both relational and physical aggression more often than boys. A report from the Bureau of Justice also found from a nationally representative sample of U.S. school-aged adolescents (ages 12–18) that girls were more frequently victimized by their peers than were boys. Moreover, girls are frequent targets of peer-to-peer sexually-based harassment, as indicated in many research findings.

In addition to the types and frequency of bullying by gender, research also shows that boys are more prone to be involved in bullying than girls, and boys may admire bullies, which might be attributed to the socially constructed view that physical aggression is symbolic of masculinity, hegemony, and power. According to Just Say Yes, boys are socialized to dominate others as a means of demonstrating their masculinity [11].

Sexual Orientation, Gender Identity, and Gender Expression

School can be an unsafe place for children and adolescents who are perceived or identified as lesbian, gay, bisexual, transgender, or "questioning" (LGBTQ. Not surprisingly, LGBTQ students are at a significant risk of being victimized by their classmates and peers in school. According to the 2015 National School Climate Survey conducted by Gay, Lesbian and Straight Education Network (GLSEN), school-aged adolescents identified as LGBTQ in middle and high schools experience hearing biased language from both students and teachers, being harassed and assaulted, being discriminated against based on sexual identity, and experience adverse educational and psychological outcomes due to a hostile school climate [12]. More specifically, the National School Climate Survey found that 27.0% of LGBTQ students reported physical harassment in the past year due to their sexual orientation, and 20.3% because of their gender. Thirteen percent were physically assaulted because of their sexual orientation and 9.4% because of their gender expression. However, 57.6% of LGBTQ students who were harassed or assaulted did not report the incident to school staff members, and of the students who reported an incident, 63.5% said the school staff did nothing in response [12]. Also, according to the report, 57.6% of LGBTQ students reported feeling unsafe in school because of their sexual orientation and 43.3% felt unsafe because of their gender identity and gender non-conformity. Homophobic bullying can be reproduced in the classrooms in many ways, including homophobic slurs, physical violence, rejection, exclusion, suppression, homophobic cyber-bullying or "outing," and creating/sharing homophobic websites. According to O'Higgins-Norman [13], *homophobic bullying* is conduct that "intentionally harasses or physically hurts another individual. It can be carried out by one person or by a group of people and it can involve direct or indirect name-calling, exclusion, mocking, or damage to a person's property. When this type of behavior arises out of the fact that the victim is identified or identifies him/herself as being gay or lesbian or if the language used in the bullying is such that it would be offensive to gay or lesbian people" [p. 6–7].

There have also been several cases of LGBTQ teens ending their own life after enduring homophobic bullying frequently in their school. Eighteen-year-old Tyler Clementi, 15-year-old Billy Lucas, and 13-year-old Asher Brown, and 13-year-old Seth Walsh are some of many students who died by *bullycide* (suicide due to bullying). On September 22, 2010, Tyler Clementi, a Rutgers University student committed suicide after his roommate secretly recorded him having sex with another man. On October 14, 2011, Jamie Hubley in Ottawa, Canada, committed suicide after years of homophobic bullying, which started in seventh grade when his classmates tried to stuff batteries in his mouth because he preferred figure skating over hockey. On August 29, 2013, a 15-year-old girl in southeast London committed suicide. Shortly before, she revealed that some people called her a lesbian or bisexual who would look at them while they were changing clothes in the gym. She had disclosed that she would cut herself every night before going to bed.

Social-Ecological Framework

In this section, we discuss the significance of sex, sexual orientation, gender identity, and gender expression in the context of bullying victimization through a social-ecological framework. More specifically, we will provide a general overview of how societal, community, institutional, group, and individual relate to bullying victimization.

Societal

As discussed in the previous section, the societal level highlights the historical, structural, and cultural factors and how they are related to bullying and peer victimization based on gender and sex differences. Factors at the societal level include social and cultural norms and values that may support bullying and violence. For instance, patriarchy, a social structure in which men possess and maintain the power, privilege, and dominant position, perpetuates oppressive gender roles, homophobia, and transphobia. Although research to date has not considered how patriarchy might reinforce bullying behavior, it is conceivable that higher rates of bullying involving boys relative to girls may be derived from patriarchy and heteronormativity, which condone aggressive behavior among boys and frame aggression as an acceptable way to resolve conflictual relationships with peers. Teenage boys are four times more likely than girls to think aggressive behavior is appropriate when someone cuts to the front of a line [14]. Moreover, under heteronormativity, same-sex sexual attraction and non-conforming gender identity are perceived as a threat to a gender norm that upholds (heterosexual) male dominance. Research has demonstrated that more rigid adherence to traditional gender roles is positively correlated with negative attitudes and violent behaviors (including bullying) toward LGBTQ youth [15, 16]. Developmentally, the association of virility and violence starts early for boys, and unlike girls, "boys do not lose their voice, they 'gain' a voice, but it is an inauthentic voice of constant posturing, of false bravado, of foolish risk-taking and gratuitous violence—what some have called the 'boy code,' the 'mask of masculinity'" [15, p. 1450]. Also, as stated by Meyer [17], "It is difficult to effectively intervene to stop bullying when the qualities that bullies embody are the ones that are most valued by many and demonstrate a power that is esteemed in a patriarchal society" [p. 38].

Policies, such as the *California Student Safety and Violence Prevention Act* of 2000 (AB537), the *Safe Place to Learn Act* of 2007 (AB394) and the *Student Civil Rights Act* of 2007 (SB777) have been implemented to address bullying and harassment in schools based on sex, gender, and sexual orientation. The California Student Safety and Violence Prevention Act prohibits discrimination, bullying, and harassment in schools based on sex, along with race, ethnic group identification, national origin, religion, color, or disabilities. It was later amended in 2000 by adding sexual orientation and gender identity to existing sections on bullying and harassment. Also, under state law, public schools and non-religious private schools that receive state funding are legally mandated to protect students from bullying, harassment, and discrimination based on the abovementioned characteristics. In 2011, *Seth's Law* (AB9) was signed by the California governor Jerry Brown, mandating school districts to include in its non-discrimination policy protecting enumerated groups from bullying in schools, such as gender, gender identity, and sexual orientation.

Community

At the community level, communities that are supportive of heteronormativity and male dominance can reinforce sexual bullying, homophobic bullying, sexual harassment in schools, for which girls and sexual minority youth are particularly targeted. A case example of homophobic bullying is the Columbine High School in Littleton, Colorado, as evidenced by a statement made by Evan Todd, a student who was wounded in the Columbine High School shootings: "Columbine is a clean, good place except for those rejects [Eric Harris and Dylan Klebold, the two school shooters]. Most kids didn't want them there. They were into witchcraft. They were into voodoo dolls. Sure, we teased them. But what do you expect with kids who come to school with weird hairdos and horns on their hats? It's not just jocks; the whole school's disgusted with them. They're [a] bunch of homos, grabbing each other's private parts. If you want to get rid of someone, usually, you tease 'em. So the whole school would call them homos, and when they did something sick, we'd tell them, 'You're sick and that's wrong'" [18]. Numerous studies have also documented that girls are significantly more likely than boys to be targets of sexual bullying [19], and youth identified as lesbian, gay, bisexual, and transgender are likely to be targeted for bullying if they reside in a neighborhood with higher LGBTQ assault hate crime rates [20] and with a higher rate of poverty. For instance, a study by Kosciw, Greytak, and Diaz [12] documented that sexual minority adolescents in rural and impoverished neighborhoods with lower adult educational attainment are likely to experience a hostile school environment where they are at risk of being victimized by their peers. Furthermore, youth residing in a neighborhood that is characterized by high community disorder and crimes may be at an elevated risk of sexual and homophobic bullying. Residents in communities where violence, crimes, and disorders are salient are less likely to provide social support and research also suggests that people in such communities are less likely to form ties with other residents in the neighborhood [21, 22].

Institutional

At the institutional level, institutions, such as religious organizations, can play a role in maintaining LGBTQ intolerance, which can promote bullying based on minority sexual orientation. A significant amount of research suggests that supportive religious institutions have a positive impact on LGBTQ youths' mental health and psychosocial well-being, such as lower rates of alcohol use and depressive symptoms [e.g., 23, 24]. However, religious ministry in churches that condemn and socially marginalize LGBTQ youth can reinforce homophobic bullying, as studies have shown [25, 26]. Homophobic bullying appears to be higher in faith-based schools in comparison to non-religious school districts. According to the School Report of the Stonewall [27], over half of the students in the non-religious school reported that their school said homophobic bullying was wrong; for faith-based schools, only 37% said homophobic bullying was wrong. The report also found that 26% of students in the non-religious school reported that their teacher did not address homophobic language, whereas, in faith-based schools, that figure rose to 36%. Besides, only 31% of the students in non-religious schools stated that their school responded quickly to homophobic bullying when it occurred, but that figure decreased to 24% in faith-based schools. Maher's [26] study, which explored homophobic bullying through interviews with gay and lesbian Catholic school alumni, demonstrated connections between religiosity, masculinity, and intolerance, and how the religious aspects of Catholic schools can contribute to homophobic bullying. The study found a significant percentage of males in Catholic schools expressing that violence against LGBTQ persons was acceptable. Bushman et al. [25] also reported that sanction of violence by God is positively correlated with greater aggression in students. More specifically, the study found that students who read a narrative about violent retaliation showed a greater tendency toward aggressive behavior. In another study, which qualitatively explored bullying of sexual and gender minority adolescents in Toronto, Canada, the language and ideology of "sin" and "conversion" were prominent in bullying of sexual and gender minority youth based on religion [28].

These study findings are consistent with statements made by students, such as Alexandra (17-years-of-age): "In religious education we learnt that the Bible was against anything other than heterosexuality. I was so scared. I had to teach myself everything. What we learnt in religious education about how we are viewed by our peers, teachers and parents made people terrified" [27, p. 35]. Another statement made by Ainsley (16 years old) also depicts how homophobic bullying is prominent in religious organizations: "It was very difficult coming out to my friends because I was not sure how they would react. Eventually over 5 years I have come out to almost everyone. The only people that don't know are people in my church because they will not accept me" [27, p. 24].

Group

Bullying is regarded as a group phenomenon and understanding group dynamics has presented challenges for schools in addressing bullying. Theoretically, social identity theory and social rules theory can explain how students reinforce the formation of "in-groups" and "out-groups," which can be breeding groups for group-based bullying. Several studies have examined the group process of gender-based bullying. In terms of gender, boys and girls may play different roles in the group process of bullying, as one study findings suggested that bullying is somewhat more related to social group dynamics in girls than in boys [29]. According to an earlier study, which included self- and peer-reports, findings suggest that girls are more likely to play the roles of defender and outsider whereas boys were more likely to assume the role of bully, reinforcer, and assistant [30]. Another study, which included self-reports, found that girls were more likely to be identified as uninvolved, whereas boys were more likely to be classified in the bully, victim, and bully/victim cluster [31]. Also, a gender difference in empathy has been implicated in research on bullying. *Empathy* is defined as "an affective response that stems from the apprehension or comprehension of another's emotional state or condition" [32, p. 316]. Empathy involves having the ability to take another's perspective or displaying feelings of compassion toward another [33]. Among the extant research, many studies have found that the association between empathy and bullying was more significant for girls than boys in group bullying situations [34], as girls tend to score higher in empathy scores than boys [35–37]. According to one longitudinal study, which explored whether females are more empathetic than males, the findings suggest that empathic response is higher in females than in males [38]. However, one study did find that low affective empathy was associated with bullying behaviors in males but not in females [39]. Moreover, studies have found that girls are significantly more likely to be peer group supporters of victims in bullying situations [e.g., 40].

We should also mention that the relationship between bullying and empathy is a complex phenomenon, which varies across gender. To illustrate, a study by Veenstra, Lindenberg, Munniksma, and Dijkstra [41] reported that bullies were rejected only by their peers to whom they represented a potential threat. For instance, male students bullying females were rejected by female classmates only; on the other hand, males targeting other males were disliked by other males but accepted by females. Another study, which presented storyboards containing bullying scenarios to 80 ten-year-old children, also found that a greater level of empathy was achieved when the characters in the scenarios were of the same gender as the child [42].

Individual

At the individual level, bullying based on sex, gender, sexual orientation, and gender identity can be fostered or inhibited by biological traits, such as biological sex and race/ethnicity. In terms of biological sex, homophobic bullying, language, and attitudes are found to be disproportionately reinforced by male students [43] and heterosexual-identified male students are frequently the targets of homophobic slurs [44]. To illustrate, an overwhelming majority of the random school shootings have been perpetrated by heterosexual-identified boys who reportedly been humiliated relentlessly with homophobic remarks by their classmates in school [45]. As Klein [46] purported, it is not simply bullying that is a precursor of school rampages, but relentless, homophobic bullying in which the school shooters "feel driven to avenge the 'wrong' and re-assert a more dominant, powerful, and victorious masculinity" [p. 39]. These findings suggest that homophobic bullying is a part of boys' gender role socialization into heteronormative and masculine attitudes, behaviors, and dispositions in a school environment that enforces a rigid system of gendered behavior [44]. As postulated by Killian and Johnson's [47] "not-me identity" concept, in schools, boys attempt to prove themselves as men by applying homophobic labels to other boys, which makes them immune to the label and solidifies their own identity as a "male."

Regarding race/ethnicity, there remains a paucity of studies that explored the intersection of race/ethnicity and sexual orientation and how it is related to gender-based or homophobic bullying, although sexual minorities of color are likely to experience dual-levels of stigma and victimization due to both their race/ethnicity and their sexual orientation [48]. Thus, there may be important racial/ethnic variations to consider in our understanding of homophobic and gender-based bullying. Such intersections can shape how adolescents of color perceive and navigate their social environment and how they experience homophobic bullying [43]. Although psychosocial outcomes of homophobic bullying have been well-documented in the research literature, there is a sparse, yet growing studies on the intersections of race/ethnicity, gender, and sexuality and bullying victimization. According to the National School Climate Survey of GLSEN in 2011, African American LGBT students were less likely to be physically or verbally harassed because of their sexual orientation, relative to their White, Hispanic, or multiracial LGBT counterparts, although 54% felt unsafe in their school because of their sexuality [49]. Other studies found that White and Hispanic LGBT youth reported skipping school because they felt unsafe [50, 51]. According to Mueller et al. [50], White and Hispanic gay and bisexual boys, White lesbian and bisexual girls, and Hispanic bisexual girls were more at risk of homophobic bullying than were White heterosexual adolescents.

Complexities

Several complexities should be considered when examining bullying based on biological sex, sexual orientation, gender expression, and gender identities. Concerning biological sex, several past studies have reported that boys are more likely to be involved in school bullying and display aggressive behavior than girls [see 52, for a review]. Moreover, other studies have found that boys engage in direct forms of bullying, whereas girls are involved in indirect forms of bullying, such as relational aggression. Scholars have questioned whether boys are indeed more aggressive than girls because past studies have excluded girls from the sample [53] and have defined aggression as overtly physical or verbal exclusively [54]. An increasing number of studies more recently found no gender differences in bullying involvement [e.g., 55, 56], which seems to suggest that both boys and girls are at risk of all types of school bullying and victimization. A seminal work by Espelage, Mebane, and Swearer [57] argued that although a tremendous amount of research addressed whether boys are more aggressive than girls, there needs to be more research that would support a response to "it depends" [58]. Although studies have documented that boys are at a significantly higher risk of engaging in bullying and being victimized, recent studies have also found that girls are significantly more likely than boys to be at risk of sexual bullying victimization at school, including sexually-based jokes, insults, and gestures; unwanted sexual attention; sexual touching; and sexual coercion [59, 60, which suggest that measures of bullying need to be seriously considered and gender-specific].

Research on homophobic bullying and violence directed at youth identified as LGBTQ in school has emerged over the years, which seems to suggest that homophobic bullying is a serious concern in American school districts. Over the past several years, we have heard many tragic stories of young people ending their lives due to homophobic bullying. Tyler Clementi, Eric Mohat, Carl Joseph Walker-Hoover, Jaheem Herrera, Billy Lucas, and Jadin Bell are just some of a countless number of young people who were reportedly bullied in school due to actual or perceived minority sexual orientation and ended their lives as a result [61]. In this chapter, we discussed the social-ecological context of homophobic bullying and how it is influenced or moderated by factors at the societal, community, institutional, group, and individual levels. We mentioned that only a handful of empirical studies take into account intersecting social identities of adolescents and how they might increase the risk of homophobic bullying. The study cited described the prevalence of racial and ethnic minorities LGBTQ youths' risk of homophobic bullying experiences [50, 51]. It is apparent that further studies are needed to disentangle the complexities of intersecting identities and how they might increase or decrease the risk of homophobic bullying. Future research on homophobic bullying might build on the existing studies by exploring how cultural factors common among racial and ethnic minorities (e.g., an obligation to the family, patriarchal family structure, and sense of machismo) might be associated with experiences in homophobic bullying and internalized homophobia among racial and ethnic minority LGBTQ adolescents. It is safe to assert that due to double minority status, racial and ethnic minority LGBTQ adolescents are at a heightened risk of homophobic bullying in their racial and ethnic communities. In a similar vein, because of their racial and ethnic minority status, these adolescents may also be racially bullied and victimized in the gay community, which is predominantly represented by white people.

Moreover, youth identified as transgender and gender non-conforming are particularly at risk of teasing, social exclusion, and violence in school due to their physical appearance, prejudiced attitudes toward transgender or gender non-conforming individuals, and socially enforced heteronormativity. Transgender and gender non-conforming adolescents may also be at a significantly higher risk of violence in school, especially as the recent administration made a sweeping decision to rescind federal guidelines to ensure protection for transgender students in public school districts. According to a GLSEN report, 75% of transgender students reported feeling unsafe at school and are highly likely to miss school out of fear for their safety. Also, according to the National Gay and Lesbian Task Force and National Center for Transgender Equality, more than half of transgender and gender non-conforming individuals who were bullied or assaulted in school have attempted suicide [62]. However, there is only a handful of research on the experiences of school bullying of adolescents identified as transgender [63, 64] and those who are gender non-conforming [65].

Conclusion

Although we attempted to explore how sex, sexual orientation, gender identity, and gender expression are related to school bullying, there is much more research needed to sufficiently understand and address bullying experiences of sexual and gender minority youth whose experiences are embedded in societal, institutional, community, peer, and individual contexts in the United States. While we have examined literature highlighting some of the ways these contexts might increase the risk of bullying of these adolescents, we argue that additional research needs to also investigate the protective factors among these groups by taking into account the complexities of intersecting identities. In addition to identifying these factors, we strongly emphasize the need to develop sex- and gender-appropriate prevention and intervention programs to address bias-based bullying in schools, which can promote academic competence. Finally, we would like to remind the reader that factors raised in this chapter about sex, sexuality, and gender and school bullying can also intersect with other identities, such as socioeconomic and social status, race and ethnicity, nationality, religious affiliation, and disabilities and special health needs.

References

1. Berlan, E. D., Corliss, H. L., Field, A. E., Goodman, E., & Austin, S. B. (2010). Sexual orientation and bullying among adolescents in the growing up today study. *Journal of Adolescent Health, 46*(4), 366–371.
2. Bontempo, D. E., & d'Augelli, A. R. (2002). Effects of at-school victimization and sexual orientation on lesbian, gay, or bisexual youths' health risk behavior. *Journal of Adolescent Health, 30*(5), 364–374.
3. Carbone-Lopez, K., Esbensen, F.-A., & Brick, B. T. (2010). Correlates and consequences of peer victimization: Gender differences in direct and indirect forms of bullying. *Youth Violence and Juvenile Justice, 8*(4), 332–350.
4. Crick, N. R., & Grotpeter, J. K. (1995). Relational aggression, gender, and social-psychological adjustment. *Child Development, 66*(3), 710–722.
5. Chapell, M. S., Hasselman, S. L., Kitchin, T., Lomon, S. N., MacIver, K. W., & Sarullo, P. L. (2006). Bullying in elementary school, high school, and college. *Adolescence, 41*(164), 633–649.
6. Griezel, L., Finger, L. R., Bodkin-Andrews, G. H., Craven, R. G., & Yeung, A. S. (2012). Uncovering the structure of and gender and developmental differences in cyber bullying. *The Journal of Educational Research, 105*(6), 442–455.
7. Hoertel, N., Le Strat, Y., Lavaud, P., & Limosin, F. (2012). Gender effects in bullying: Results from a national sample. *Psychiatry Research, 200*(2–3), 921–927.
8. Silva, M. A., Pereira, B., Mendonça, D., Nunes, B., & Oliveira, W. A. d. (2013). The involvement of girls and boys with bullying: An analysis of gender differences. *International Journal of Environmental Research and Public Health, 10*(12), 6820–6831.
9. Hong, J. S. (2009). Feasibility of the Olweus bullying prevention program in low-income schools. *Journal of School Violence, 8*(1), 81–97.
10. Putallaz, M., Grimes, C. L., Foster, K. J., Kupersmidt, J. B., Coie, J. D., & Dearing, K. (2007). Overt and relational aggression and victimization: Multiple perspectives within the school setting. *Journal of School Psychology, 45*(5), 523–547.

11. Covington, M. (n.d.). Brutal Boys versus Mean Girls - Just Say YES Anti-Bullying Programs. Retrieved August 18, 2020, from https://www.justsayyes.org/bullying/brutal-boys-vs-mean-girls/
12. Kosciw, J., Greytak, E., Giga, N., Villenas, C., & Danischewski, D. (2015). The 2015 School Climate Survey: The experiences of lesbian, gay, bisexual, transgender, and queer youth in our nation's schools. New York: GLSEN. Retrieved May 15, 2017. https://www.glsen.org/sites/default/files/2015%20National%20GLSEN%202015%20National%20School%20Climate%20Survey%20%28NSCS%29%20-%20Full%20Report_0.pdf
13. O'Higgins-Norman, J. (2008). *Homophobic bullying in Irish secondary education*. Palo Alto, CA: Academic Press.
14. Kimmel, M. S. (2000). *The gendered society*. New York: Oxford University Press.
15. Bufkin, J. L. (1999). Bias crime as gendered behavior. *Social Justice, 26*(1), 155–176.
16. Whitley, B. E. (2001). Gender-role variables and attitudes toward homosexuality. *Sex Roles, 45*(11–12), 691–721.
17. Meyer, E. (2008). A feminist reframing of bullying and harassment: Transforming schools through critical pedagogy. *McGill Journal of Education/Revue des sciences de l'éducation de McGill, 43*(1), 33–48.
18. Gibbs, N., Roche, T., & Goldstein, A. (1999). The columbine tapes. *Time, 154*(25), 40–51.
19. Shute, R., Owens, L., & Slee, P. (2008). Everyday victimization of adolescent girls by boys: Sexual harassment, bullying or aggression? *Sex Roles, 58*(7–8), 477–489.
20. Hatzenbuehler, M. L., Duncan, D., & Johnson, R. (2015). Neighborhood-level LGBT hate crimes and bullying among sexual minority youths: A geospatial analysis. *Violence and Victims, 30*(4), 663–675.
21. Ross, C. E., & Mirowsky, J. (2009). Neighborhood disorder, subjective alienation, and distress. *Journal of Health and Social Behavior, 50*(1), 49–64.
22. Sampson, R. J., Morenoff, J. D., & Gannon-Rowley, T. (2002). Assessing "neighborhood effects": Social processes and new directions in research. *Annual Review of Sociology, 28*(1), 443–478.
23. Gattis, M. N., Woodford, M. R., & Han, Y. (2014). Discrimination and depressive symptoms among sexual minority youth: Is gay-affirming religious affiliation a protective factor? *Archives of Sexual Behavior, 43*(8), 1589–1599.
24. Hatzenbuehler, M. L., Pachankis, J. E., & Wolff, J. (2012). Religious climate and health risk behaviors in sexual minority youths: A population-based study. *American Journal of Public Health, 102*(4), 657–663.
25. Bushman, B. J., Ridge, R. D., Das, E., Key, C. W., & Busath, G. L. (2007). When god sanctions killing: Effect of scriptural violence on aggression. *Psychological Science, 18*(3), 204–207.
26. Maher, M. J. (2013). Homophobic bullying in Catholic high schools: Five US studies in heterosexism, authority, masculinity, and religion. In Z. Gross, L. Davies, & A. K. Diab (Eds.), *Gender, religion and education in a chaotic postmodern world* (pp. 271–284). Dordrecht: Springer.
27. Bradlow, J., Bartram, F., Guasp, A., & Jadva, V. (2017). *School report: The experiences of lesbian, gay, bi and trans young people in Britain's schools in 2017*. London: Stonewall.
28. Newman, P. A., Fantus, S., Woodford, M. R., & Rwigema, M.-J. (2018). "Pray that God will change you": The religious social ecology of bias-based bullying targeting sexual and gender minority youth—A qualitative study of service providers and educators. *Journal of Adolescent Research, 33*(5), 523–548.
29. Crapanzano, A. M., Frick, P. J., Childs, K., & Terranova, A. M. (2011). Gender differences in the assessment, stability, and correlates to bullying roles in middle school children. *Behavioral Sciences & the Law, 29*(5), 677–694.
30. Salmivalli, C. (2010). Bullying and the peer group: A review. *Aggression and Violent Behavior, 15*(2), 112–120.
31. Espelage, D. L., & Holt, M. K. (2007). Dating violence & sexual harassment across the bully-victim continuum among middle and high school students. *Journal of Youth and Adolescence, 36*(6), 799–811.

32. Eisenberg, N., & Liew, J. (n.d.). Empathy. In R. A. Shweder, T. R. Bidell, A. C. Dailey, S. D. Dixon, P. J. Miller, & J. Modell (Eds.), *The child: An encyclopedic companion* (pp. 316–318). Chicago, IL: University of Chicago Press.
33. Davis, M. H. (1983). Measuring individual differences in empathy: Evidence for a multidimensional approach. *Journal of Personality and Social Psychology, 44*(1), 113.
34. Jolliffe, D., & Farrington, D. P. (2006). Examining the relationship between low empathy and bullying. *Aggressive Behavior, 32*(6), 540–550.
35. Del Rey, R., Lazuras, L., Casas, J. A., Barkoukis, V., Ortega-Ruiz, R., & Tsorbatzoudis, H. (2016). Does empathy predict (cyber) bullying perpetration, and how do age, gender and nationality affect this relationship? *Learning and Individual Differences, 45*, 275–281.
36. Landazabal, M. G. (2009). A comparative analysis of empathy in childhood and adolescence: Gender differences and associated socio-emotional variables. *International Journal of Psychology and Psychological Therapy, 9*(2), 217–235.
37. Van Noorden, T. H., Haselager, G. J., Cillessen, A. H., & Bukowski, W. M. (2015). Empathy and involvement in bullying in children and adolescents: A systematic review. *Journal of Youth and Adolescence, 44*(3), 637–657.
38. Mestre Escriva, M. V., Samper, P., Frías, M. D., & Tur, A. M. (2009). Are women more empathetic than men? A longitudinal study in adolescence. Spanish Journal of Psychology, 12, 76–83. Retrieved from http://redalyc.uaemex.mx/redalyc/pdf/172/17213005008.pdf.
39. Jolliffe, D., & Farrington, D. P. (2011). Is low empathy related to bullying after controlling for individual and social background variables? Journal of Adolescence, 34(1), 59–71.
40. Cowie, H. (2000). Bystanding or standing by: Gender issues in coping with bullying in English schools. *Aggressive Behavior, 26*(1), 85–97.
41. Veenstra, R., Lindenberg, S., Munniksma, A., & Dijkstra, J. K. (2010). The complex relation between bullying, victimization, acceptance, and rejection: Giving special attention to status, affection, and sex differences. *Child Development, 81*(2), 480–486.
42. Woods, S., Hall, L., Dautenhahn, K., & Wolke, D. (2007). Implications of gender differences for the development of animated characters for the study of bullying behavior. *Computers in Human Behavior, 23*(1), 770–786.
43. Poteat, V. P., & Rivers, I. (2010). The use of homophobic language across bullying roles during adolescence. *Journal of Applied Developmental Psychology, 31*(2), 166–172.
44. Pascoe, C. J. (2011). *Dude, you're a fag: Masculinity and sexuality in high school*. University of California Press.
45. The New York Times (1999). The community: Columbine students talk of the disaster and life. Retrieved August 18, 2020, from https://archive.nytimes.com/www.nytimes.com/library/national/043099colo-voices.html
46. Klein, J. (2006). Sexuality and school shootings: What role does teasing play in school massacres? *Journal of Homosexuality, 51*(4), 39–62.
47. Killian, C., & Johnson, C. (2006). "I'm not an immigrant!": Resistance, redefinition, and the role of resources in identity work. *Social Psychology Quarterly, 69*(1), 60–80.
48. Hightow-Weidman, L. B., Phillips, G., Jones, K. C., Outlaw, A. Y., Fields, S. D., Smith, J. C., & for The YMSM of Color SPNS Initiative Study Group. (2011). Racial and sexual identity-related maltreatment among minority YMSM: Prevalence, perceptions, and the association with emotional distress. *AIDS Patient Care and STDs, 25*(S1), S39–S45.
49. Kosciw, J. G., Greytak, E. A., Bartkiewicz, M. J., Boesen, M. J., & Palmer, N. A. (2012). *The 2011 National School Climate Survey: The experiences of lesbian, gay, bisexual and transgender youth in our nation's schools*. ERIC.
50. Mueller, A. S., James, W., Abrutyn, S., & Levin, M. L. (2015). Suicide ideation and bullying among US adolescents: Examining the intersections of sexual orientation, gender, and race/ethnicity. *American Journal of Public Health, 105*(5), 980–985.
51. Russell, S. T., Everett, B. G., Rosario, M., & Birkett, M. (2014). Indicators of victimization and sexual orientation among adolescents: Analyses from youth risk behavior surveys. *American Journal of Public Health, 104*(2), 255–261.

52. Archer, J. (2004). Sex differences in aggression in real-world settings: A meta-analytic review. *Review of General Psychology, 8*(4), 291–322.
53. Card, N. A., & Little, T. D. (2006). Proactive and reactive aggression in childhood and adolescence: A meta-analysis of differential relations with psychosocial adjustment. *International Journal of Behavioral Development, 30*(5), 466–480.
54. Espelage, D. L., & Swearer, S. M. (2003). Research on school bullying and victimization: What have we learned and where do we go from here? *School Psychology Review, 32*(3), 365–383.
55. Barboza, G. E., Schiamberg, L. B., Oehmke, J., Korzeniewski, S. J., Post, L. A., & Heraux, C. G. (2009). Individual characteristics and the multiple contexts of adolescent bullying: An ecological perspective. *Journal of Youth and Adolescence, 38*(1), 101–121.
56. Lansford, J. E., Skinner, A. T., Sorbring, E., Giunta, L. D., Deater-Deckard, K., Dodge, K. A., et al. (2012). Boys' and girls' relational and physical aggression in nine countries. Aggressive Behavior, 38(4), 298–308.
57. Espelage, D. L., Mebane, S. E., & Swearer, S. M. (2004). Gender differences in bullying: Moving beyond mean level differences. In D. L. Espelage & S. M. Swearer (Eds.), *Bullying in American schools* (pp. 15–35). Mahwah, NJ: Erlbaum.
58. Knight, G. P., Guthrie, I. K., Page, M. C., & Fabes, R. A. (2002). Emotional arousal and gender differences in aggression: A meta-analysis. *Aggressive Behavior, 28*(5), 366–393.
59. Lipson, J. (2001). *Hostile hallways: Bullying, teasing, and sexual harassment in school*. ERIC.
60. Hand, J. Z., & Sanchez, L. (2000). Badgering or bantering? Gender differences in experience of, and reactions to, sexual harassment among US high school students. *Gender & Society, 14*(6), 718–746.
61. Pascoe, C. J. (2013). Notes on a sociology of bullying: Young men's homophobia as gender socialization. *QED: A Journal in GLBTQ Worldmaking*, 87–104.
62. National Center for Transgender Equality (2010). Bullying, Transgender Students and the Risk of Suicide. Retrieved August 18, 2020, from https://myemail.constantcontact.com/Bullying%2D%2DTransgender-Students-and-the-Risk-of-Suicide.html?soid=1100409733839&aid=uKN5iQ_U6L4
63. Goldblum, P., Testa, R. J., Pflum, S., Hendricks, M. L., Bradford, J., & Bongar, B. (2012). The relationship between gender-based victimization and suicide attempts in transgender people. *Professional Psychology: Research and Practice, 43*(5), 468.
64. Ybarra, M. L., Mitchell, K. J., & Kosciw, J. (2014). The relation between suicidal ideation and bullying victimization in a national sample of transgender and non-transgender adolescents. In D. L. Espelage, J. Chu, & B. Bongar (Eds.), *Youth suicide and bullying: Challenges and strategies for prevention and intervention* (pp. 134–147). New York, NY: Oxford University Press.
65. Aspenlieder, L., Buchanan, C. M., McDougall, P., & Sippola, L. K. (2009). Gender nonconformity and peer victimization in pre-and early adolescence. *International Journal of Developmental Science, 3*(1), 3–16.

Chapter 6
The Color of School Bullying Victimization: Race, Ethnicity, Immigration, and Religion

Abstract In this chapter, we explain how race, ethnicity, immigration, and religion are associated with school bullying. Most school bullying research has focused on the differential patterns of victimization between White American and African American youth. Research reveals that African American, Latino American, Asian American, and White American youth experience school bullying victimization distinctly differently. We discuss several potential reasons have why racial and ethnic minority youth have increased exposure to school bullying. Immigrant youth are also often subjected to negative treatment such as discrimination, ridicule, and harassment from other students, teachers, and school administrators. Moreover, perceptions of low academic ability, rejection by peers, and fear of safety are all reflective of immigrant youth experiences within the United States school system. Additionally, the events of September 11, 2001, resulted in a dramatic increase in the religious-based bullying victimization, harassment, verbal and physical threats toward youth who are or are perceived to be Muslim in school.

Keywords Race and ethnicity · Immigration · Religion

Introduction

In this chapter, we explore how race, ethnicity, immigration, and religion are relevant to school bullying. Most school bullying research has focused on the differential patterns of victimization between White American and Black/African American youth. Research, however, suggests significant differences among different racial and ethnic groups. We first discuss how racial and ethnic disparities are related to bullying victimization in U.S. school districts. We then present how characteristics correlated with immigration can influence the likelihood of school bullying victimization. Immigrant youth are often subjected to negative treatment, such as discrimination, ridicule, harassment, and bullying from other students, teachers, and school administrators. Next, we describe how religion can predispose youth to bullying victimization. For instance, the events of September 11, 2001, resulted in a dramatic increase in bullying victimization, harassment, verbal and physical threats toward youth identified as or perceived to be Muslim Americans in school. We then discuss

A. A. Peguero, J. S. Hong, *School Bullying*, Springer Series on Child and Family Studies, https://doi.org/10.1007/978-3-030-64367-6_6

how race, ethnicity, immigration, and religion should be considered in the phenomenon of bullying victimization through a social-ecological framework. In the final section of this chapter, we highlight the complexities associated with understanding race, ethnicity, immigration, religion, and youth victimization, and school bullying.

Race and Ethnicity

About one-third of the current U.S. youth population belongs to a racial and ethnic minority group and it is projected that racial and ethnic minorities will comprise more than half of all U.S. youth by 2025 [1]. Given that, the growth of racial and ethnic minorities will have major implications for school experiences and educational opportunities, and understanding and addressing racial and ethnic disparities in U.S. schools is imperative.

Historically, most scholars of school bullying have focused on the different patterns of victimization between Black/African American and White American students. More recently, however, an increasing number of studies have revealed clear distinctions between the likelihood of school bullying victimization for Black/African American, Latina/o American, Asian American, and White American youth. In 2015, higher percentages of Black/African American students (25%) and White American students (22%) than of Latina/o American students (17%) reported being bullied at school. The percentage of students who reported being made fun of, called names, or insulted was also higher for Black/African American students (17%) and White American students (14%) than for Latina/o American students (9%). The percentage of students who reported being the subject of rumors was higher for Black/African American students (14%), White American students (13%), and Latina/o American students (10%) than for Asian American students (5%) [2]. Although it appears that the prevalence rate of bullying victimization is lower among racial and ethnic minorities compared to White American students, research findings still report significantly high rates of bullying and victimization among these populations. For instance, findings from Low et al.'s [3] study, which comprised a sample of 2165 fourth and fifth graders in 13 elementary schools in Texas indicate that as many as 88% of Latino American students experience bullying victimization, and results from several studies document that Asian American students are more likely to experience peer victimization and social exclusion than students of other racial and ethnic groups [4, 5]. Sawyer et al. [5] also reported that Latino American and Asian American students are more likely than White American students to report experiencing all forms of victimization in their school.

In the changing racial and ethnic demographic landscape within the United States and its schools, bullying victimization may contribute to the historic and persistent racial and ethnic educational gaps. The educational consequence of school bullying victimization seems to be more severe for Black/African American and Latino American students, as measured by sharper declines in grades and test scores as well as increased odds of dropping out of school [6]. Additionally, some researchers have reported that school officials' perceptions of minority youths' tolerance for bullying are higher than it is for their White American classmates [7, 8]. These studies have suggested that school officials often perceive that bullying and violence are daily aspects of racial and ethnic minority students' experiences, while exposure to violence is less frequent among White American students. The attention and concerns by school counselors, teachers, and administrators toward White American students' exposure to violence and bullying are relatively higher, in comparison to the victimization of racial and ethnic minority youth [7, 8].

Immigration

Children of immigrants are often considered to be more at risk for mistreatment, due to the stress and pressure that they and their families experience in the migration process. It is critical to point out that the immigration experience denotes a major life transition that often engenders fear, loss, isolation, confusion, and uncertainty about the present and future. Although there are countless reasons for migration, such as poverty, war, famine, religious persecution, and disaster, the process of leaving one's home, country, and culture is not an isolated event. Rather, educators should be reminded that the processes associated with migration and immigration are lengthy and difficult and can sometimes involve dangerous journeys for children and their families. Language barriers, racism, discrimination, prejudice, xenophobia, and unfamiliar customs are all part of the diverse social and cultural experiences for the children and adolescents of immigrants [9, 10].

As previously mentioned, one out of four children in U.S. school districts currently has at least one immigrant parent and this proportion is expected to rise to one in three by 2025 [1]. Contrary to societal perceptions and popular media depictions, many of the children in immigrant families were born in the United States [9, 10]., which means that many children of immigrants are, in fact, U.S. citizens. Therefore, the children of immigrants who live in the United States are legally entitled to an educational experience that is fair, equitable, and effective. However, the challenges faced by U.S. school districts concerning the children of immigrants are not new.

It is in school that the children of immigrants are exposed to mainstream American culture and where they learn and form beliefs about what U.S. society and persons outside of their families expect from them. Negative treatment by classmates, peers, and school officials, such as bullying, can further marginalize an already vulnerable population. The children of immigrants are often subjected to racism, discrimination, ridicule, and harassment from other students as well as from school staff [9, 11–13]. Perceptions of low academic ability, rejection by peers, and threats against their safety are all reflective of the children of immigrants' experiences within the U.S. school system. Teachers can sometimes present barriers to the educational success of the children of immigrants in their classrooms. Some teachers treat the children of immigrants as a burden or less capable than other students and argue that immigrant students limit their ability to teach effectively and efficiently. A few rationalizations for holding negative or unwelcoming perceptions include chronic lack of time to address the unique needs of children of immigrants, perceived intensification of teacher workloads when children of immigrants are enrolled in their classes, and feelings of social and cultural inadequacy when working with the children of immigrants. Because teachers may perceive that these children restrict advancement and educational progress for the entire class, they are sometimes reluctant to accept and effectively teach immigrant children in their classrooms. Meanwhile, children of immigrants are less likely to report victimization and discriminatory treatment because of fear of deportation for themselves or their family members, regardless of their citizenship status [11–14].

Religion

Few studies have examined the association between religious affiliation and school bullying. Religious affiliation can either be a risk or protective factor for bullying. Youth who frequently attend religious institutions may be less likely to be involved in school bullying but are more likely to be bullied and teased for their religious beliefs [8]. In other words, religiously devout youth indicate that their school experiences include being bullied by secular youth because of their religious beliefs. There is recent emerging research, however, suggesting that, after the September 11, 2001, terrorist attacks, the harassment of youth who are actual or perceived to be Muslims have been increasing, including within schools.

After the September 11, 2001, terrorist attacks, people across the United states who appeared to fit the generic mold of Arab, Muslim, or Middle Easterners (and therefore the enemy in the wider public's perception) were targets of violence [15–17]. In actuality, those targeted by this bias included a wide range of ethnic and religious groups, including Christians, Muslims, and Hindus, of Arab, Pakistani, Sikh, and Indian descent. During this period fear of harassment, violence, and victimization swept through Arab, Muslim, and South Asian communities [15–17]. The term "Islamophobia" has emerged to reflect the historical, social, and political context of the fear of Islam and Muslim Americans in the post 9–11 era. Unfortunately, Islamophobia found its way into schools.

Research has shown that Muslim American girls who wear hijabs (headscarves) and Sikh American boys who wear patka or dastaar (turbans) report being targeted because of these visible symbols of their religious heritage and the general public's misconceptions of their associations with terrorism [15–17]. Muslim American students also report being confronted with explicitly biased treatment, derogatory slurs, verbal assaults, and threats of physical violence directed at themselves as well as their families by not only students and their parents, but also by school administrators, teachers, and security personnel. In ethnographic research, Abu El-Haj [15] reported that several veiled, Muslim American female students were harassed in their school, being told by their teachers that they "look like a disgrace in that thing," while some were threatened with disciplinary sanctions if they did not remove their headscarves.

Social-Ecological Framework

In this section, we present the significance of race, ethnicity, immigration, and religion in the context of bullying victimization through a social-ecological framework. Although we will not specifically exemplify how societal, community, institutional, group, and individual behaviors relate to race, ethnicity, immigration, and religion, we will provide a general overview. Then, we will follow up with a discussion of the complexities associated with linking bullying victimization, race, ethnicity, immigration, religion, and the social-ecological framework.

Societal

At the societal level, there are harmful processes that have marginalized racial and ethnic minorities, immigrants, and religious groups, and contribute to making these populations vulnerable to bullying and violence in school. In short, historical, structural, systemic, and overarching racial and ethnic disparities in the United States are associated with school violence, victimization, and bullying.

Racial and ethnic disparities in the U.S. school system are historic, persistent, and continue to be evident [9, 18–22]. Racial and ethnic educational disparities in schools go back to the late 1880s with the emergence of public schooling: racial and ethnic minority groups were not afforded the same educational opportunities as most of their White American majority counterparts. Segregated schools were established and sustained throughout the United States to support White power and privilege as well as reinforce educational disparities. During enslavement, African Americans in the South were denied formal and informal schooling, and after the Reconstruction Era (1865–1877) they were not allowed to attend schools with White Americans. Latino Americans (primarily Mexican Americans) and Asian Americans during this time were also excluded from attending schools with White Americans. For years, federal and state laws supported separate schooling. The 1896 *Plessy v. Ferguson* Supreme Court decision upheld the practice of separate accommodations for minorities and White Americans. This case provided a legal precedent for "separate but equal" accommodations in all public institutions including schools; however, it became evident that separate schools were inherently unequal. School segregation reflected a two-tier and hierarchical educational system in which minority schools lacked the funding, physical facilities, textbooks, and supplies that the majority had enjoyed, thus ensuring that minority students were provided a poor education. The fight against legalized racial and ethnic educational segregation was pursued with *Mendez v. Westminster* (1946) and *Brown v. Board of*

Education (1954) Supreme Court cases, which led the Supreme Court to rule that segregating schools were unconstitutional and ordered that racial and ethnic segregation in schools be eliminated. This allowed racial and ethnic minorities the right to attend schools with White Americans. These landmark cases were pivotal in promoting public school integration for all racial and ethnic minority groups. However, even 60 years after these historic Supreme Court cases, U.S. schools are still significantly segregated [9, 18–22].

The persistence of U.S. racial and ethnic educational disparities is still apparent and contributes to racial and ethnic minority students' vulnerability to school violence, victimization, and harassment in fundamental ways, including limited funding and restricted access to resources. Schools with predominantly minority students are often underfunded and not adequately staffed to sustain school programs that have proven to ameliorate bullying and violence, as well as improve overall school climates. These factors directly affect the success and sustainability of anti-bullying programs, because schools serving racial and ethnic minority students receive fewer resources, face greater difficulties attracting qualified teachers, encounter many more challenges in addressing students' needs, and receive less support from communities as well as community businesses [12, 18, 19, 23].

Community

Because schools are embedded in communities, an unsafe neighborhood environment can influence youth bullying behavior as a result of a lack of adult supervision or negative peer influences. Researchers consistently find an association between community violence and bullying behavior [8, 23–25]. Youth residing in unsafe communities may reflect a larger social environment in which bullying and violence are frequent occurrences. Schools serving predominately racial and ethnic minority students are often embedded in urban communities with higher levels of poverty, unemployment, crime, and violence [7, 25–28]. Studies also indicate that the development of social ties to conventional institutions and belief in conventional values becomes problematic for residents living in such communities. Therefore, social conditions in these communities can make it challenging for racial and ethnic minority youth to form strong bonds (e.g., attachment, commitment, involvement, and belief) with conventional social institutions, such as schools. In other words, racial and ethnic minority youth are more likely to have weaker social bonds to conventional institutions and therefore are more likely to be involved in delinquency and violence in their communities and schools [24–30]. Weak social bonds to school are also associated with an increase in student's misbehavior and bullying within the school. Students who are well integrated, connected, attached, involved, and committed to school are more likely to obey and follow the rules and refrain from misbehaviors such as bullying. This is particularly relevant because racial and ethnic minority youth are often socialized to believe, through overt and subtle ways, that being a minority means having less power in society, being discriminated against, having fewer economic and educational opportunities, and being perceived as potential troublemakers, as well as being a burden upon society by social institutions including schools [24–30].

In Elijah Anderson's [26] seminal work, *Code of the Street*, he argues that the disproportionate levels of violence within minority communities result from high rates of poverty, joblessness, alienation, mistrust of police, and hopelessness. In turn, to survive in this situation, racial and ethnic minority youth often incorporate an oppositional culture that rejects mainstream values. Anderson refers to this oppositional culture as the "code of the street." The code of the street emphasizes garnering the respect of others through a violent identity and toughness. As a result, minority youth who are "tough" does not get disrespected, victimized, and bullied. Research suggests that these alienated youth, who view their communities and schools as plagued by social problems and disorder, may develop a social identity as individuals who engage in violence and bullying, as a way to deflect or avoid being victimized [26–29, 31]. Additionally, because the schools that these youth attend often have increased levels of disorder, it seems consistent with previous research that school misbehavior and bullying by some racial and ethnic minority youth may be viewed as a strategy used to reduce the risk of being victimized.

There is considerable overlap between the community and school youth interactions that can contribute to bullying and violence. It is often reported that the many incidents of school-related violence affecting minority youth occur on the way to school, beyond school grounds or immediately following school hours [24, 27, 28, 30, 31]. Because schools, especially high schools, can draw students from a larger community area, strong territorial identities associated with youth gangs can contribute to increased contact and potential conflict among racial and ethnic minority youth with one another while entering and exiting school grounds.

Institutional

At the institutional level, school practices or processes may be contributing to the marginalization of racial and ethnic minorities. For example, threats can perpetuate or reproduce oppression, marginalization, and privilege based on race, ethnicity, immigration, and/or religion, which can undermine youth's educational success and social progress and increase vulnerability to bullying and violence.

The perspective of examining school as a place where students compete for educational resources and opportunities for success are both historical and current [9, 18–20, 32]. Therefore, feeling threatened can influence individuals to act in ways that protect their interests, even using violence. The increase in the size of minority populations, including within schools, increases the perceptions of threat and competition for economic and educational resources and opportunities. Research finds that, as racial and ethnic minority student population increases in schools, so do parents' decisions to move residences or to change their children to another school. Historically battles over bussing have ensued, along with stringent discipline practices, ability grouping, and tracking [32, 33]. It is plausible that these school practices or processes can fuel bullying and aggression among racial and ethnic minority youth groups within schools because they view each other as threats, perceiving that education is a zero-sum game, with the need to defend educational resources and opportunities along with academic self-interests.

The social and political debates around U.S. immigration policy are heated and controversial. Much of the argument is centered on the myth that increasing levels of immigration contributes to increased crime, higher levels of unemployment, greater likelihood of abuse of public service resources, and diminished educational opportunities [9, 10, 34–36]. The perceived threat of immigration vilifying immigrants and their children, when it seeps into schools can foster aggression, bullying, and violence directed toward immigrant students. Perceptions of low academic ability, peer rejection, discrimination, harassment, bullying, and fear of safety are all reflective of the children of immigrants' reports of their school experiences [10–14, 34, 35, 37]. A few "rationalizations" that school administrators, teachers, parents, and students have for holding negative or unwelcoming views include the chronic lack of time to address the unique needs of the children of immigrants, perceived intensification of teacher workloads when the children of immigrants are enrolled in their classes, and feelings of professional inadequacy to work with immigrant children [9, 10, 34, 35]. School personnel can be reluctant to accept, have, keep, and teach the children of immigrants in their schools and classrooms. For instance, in 2011, Alabama Governor Robert Bentley signed House Bill 56, which mandated school practices or processes to verify the citizenship of students and inform police about families who don't have proper identification. Consequently, there have been increased reports of the children of immigrants being threatened with deportation by other students and school personnel.

The events of September 11, 2001, resulted in a dramatic increase in the bullying victimization, harassment, verbal and physical threats toward Muslim youth in U.S. schools [15–17]. Since that tragedy, the rhetoric and political climate threatening Muslim Americans, or Islamophobia, fueled hate crimes against Muslim Americans. A peak of the U.S. anti-Muslim sentiment was evidenced by the backlash against the building of an Islamic youth center "near" Ground Zero in New York City and the Florida pastor who gained worldwide attention by threatening to burn dozens of Qurans. The threat against Muslims certainly found its way into schools. Muslim American students were subjected to many forms of harassment including mockery, as well as physical violence, and even death threats, not only from other students but from teachers as well [15–17]. U.S. schools decree that all students are to be treated equally, that all children are to be given the same mainstream curricula, and that all students are to behave and respond to schools' practices in the same way, regardless of culture or religion [15–17]. In this way, schools become key places where dominant American cultures and values are transmitted and where the freedom to express and practice minority cultures or values, such as those of Islam, is resisted.

Group

Schools are composed of groups of individuals in a setting with whom youth have daily interactions. This level examines the close relationships that may increase the risk of violent victimization or perpetration. A youth's closest social circle-peers at school could contribute to their odds of being bullied and victimized. In relationship to race and ethnicity, some argue that stereotypes can foster aggression, bullying, and peer conflicts between and among school peers of distinct racial and ethnic backgrounds.

Stereotypes are judgments of individuals, which are based on their membership in specific social groups [38, 39]. In everyday social settings, observers treat information about social category membership (e.g., racial and ethnic minority groups) as a guide to an actor's behavioral, physical, and psychological attributes. Such information may engender subjective attitudes and influence social perceptions, evaluative judgments, and stereotypes made by and about individuals. Children learn to become aware of race and ethnicity as social categories at an early age. By the age of three, children label themselves and others according to race and ethnicity [38, 39]. Among the more pervasive inferences drawn by and about children based on their racial and ethnic group identification are inferences that assume individual differences in academic performances, behaviors related to achievement, and motivation for schooling [38, 39]. Consequently, within schools, perceived racial and ethnic differences may reinforce stereotypes about the appropriate behaviors and social roles for individuals from certain racial and ethnic backgrounds. For instance, Black/African Americans and Latino Americans often are stereotyped as being poor, limited in their academic potential, and having superior physical and athletic abilities. In contrast, Asian Americans are stereotyped as "model minorities" who achieve universal and unparalleled academic success but possess limited physical and athletic abilities [9, 38].

Thus, Black/African American, Latino American, and Asian American youth who do not conform to these stereotypes often face resistance, verbal harassment, derogatory treatment, and social isolation from their classmates and peers of all racial and ethnic backgrounds. In other words, there are intra- and inter-racial and ethnic tensions between minority youth who do not match these stereotypes and their peers [6, 38]. To illustrate, Black/African American youth who achieve academic success are perceived by their peers as "acting White" [40]. These findings suggest that there are repercussions or a "backlash" for racial and ethnic minorities who go against the stereotypes. Rudman and Fairchild [39] proposed a conceptual framework that predicted backlash in stereotype maintenance from the perspective of both perceivers and actors. Cultural stereotypes reinforce a normative standard to which the target is compared; when individuals do not conform to the standard, a contrast effect may cause them to be perceived as deviant [39]. In turn, "backlash effects" allowed perceivers to feel justified (e.g., when they feel threatened or desire revenge). Bullying victimization may be a form of backlash against those who do not conform to the socially constructed racial and ethnic stereotypes; that is, Black/

African American, Latino American, and Asian American youth who do not conform to the racial and ethnic stereotypes may be more likely at risk of bullying victimization.

Individual

Individual violence and bullying encompass behavior that focuses on individual youth at school. The defining characteristic of bullying at this level involves the individual's vulnerability to being bullied while on the way to, from, or at school. In relationship to race and ethnicity, immigration, and religion, some argue that a youth's routines and activities can influence their vulnerability to being bullied and victimized.

Routine Activity Theory focuses on the circumstances surrounding violent events, rather than the motivation of offenders. For victimization to occur, there must be a convergence in time and space of motivated offenders, suitable targets, and the absence of capable guardians [13, 30, 41]. Research demonstrates that exposure to bullying, victimization, and violence varies by a youth's school activities and routines. For instance, youths' participation in extracurricular activities such as school government, band, clubs, and sports should protect them because of the number of adults present. Wilcox, Tillyer, and Fisher [41] suggest, "even though structured before- and after-school activities are supervised by adults, the relative amount of supervision available can be much less than during normal school hours (i.e., hallways, locker rooms, etc.) are typically left unattended while extracurricular activities are ongoing in particular areas of the school or grounds)" [p. 248]. Therefore, participation in extracurricular activities may contribute to distinct vulnerabilities for school bullying victimization. Although a youth's routines and activities can be associated with the likelihood of being bullied and victimized on the way to or at school, there is evidence indicating that factors of race, ethnicity, immigration, or religion can moderate the relationship between school routines and activities and bullying victimization.

Racial and ethnic minority youth often reside in neighborhoods and attend schools located in their neighborhood that have higher concentrations of crime and disorder, exposing them to potentially higher rates of violence, both directly and indirectly, on their way to school. Thus, it is not surprising that racial and ethnic minority youth report being more afraid of being victimized on their way to school than White American youth [29]. Who is perceived as a "suitable target" is related to a youth's involvement in academic and/or sport school activities. A youth's participation in academics (e.g., band, government, newspaper, etc.) and/or sport school activities varies by racial and ethnic groups, therefore the relationship between target suitability and victimization would also vary by race and ethnicity [38, 42]. Participation in academic school activities is a potential risk factor for victimization exclusively for racial and ethnic minorities. Moreover, engagement in school sports is a potential risk factor for victimization among Latino American and Asian American youth [38, 42].

As already noted in this chapter, immigrant families face a myriad of challenges, such as residing in communities with high levels of poverty, unwelcoming receptions, discrimination and biased treatment, and community violence exposure, all of which results in children of immigrants, directly and indirectly, being vulnerable to violence and victimization on their way to school. Also, research demonstrates that children of immigrants also navigate through their routines or route to and from school to avoid victimization and harassment because potential offenders are aware that the children of immigrants are afraid of reporting their victimization [11–13, 37]. Peguero [13] finds that target suitability is linked to school-based victimization for the children of immigrants. He notes that the children of immigrants' levels and types of school-based activities are distinct. These children are less likely to engage in extracurricular activities because their language, cultural, and social barriers make it difficult to engage in academic, sport, and club school activities. These factors make their relationship between school routines and bullying victimization distinct among children of immigrants.

From the standpoint of religion, considering the ways that Muslims American youth are visible in U.S. society, it is not surprising that these youth often find themselves confronting negative, inaccurate, and monolithic images of their cultural or religious practices on their way to, from, and at school [15–17]. In response to what they experience as a pervasive climate of ignorance about or hostility toward being Muslim, there are distinct routines and activities these children adopt to navigate and avoid being bullied, victimized, and harassed. In practicing their Islamic faith, certain customs and activities are expected, for example, adhering to religious dress (for girls), prayer time, and fasting during Ramadan. Basford [16] expresses that Muslim American youth encounter religious discrimination and ignorance at school, which influences their school routines and activities. She cites an example of when Muslim American youth participated in a school book club exchange, they heard students often yell "there go the little terrorists" and observed several people in the math class, including the math teacher, laugh loudly as the Muslim American youth engaged in this school activity [16]. Besides, some Muslim American youth need to find random places to pray such as "between classrooms, in the hallways, in the music hall...anywhere [they] could find a place," which often results in being bullied and harass before, during, and after prayers [16, p. 496].

Complexities

Several complexities should be considered when trying to understand how race, ethnicity, immigration, and religion are associated with school bullying. In relationship to race and ethnicity, in this chapter, we have focused on pan-ethnic terms. For instance, extant research on youth victimization and school bullying among Latino American and Asian American youth have not considered the cultural differences among particular racial and ethnic subgroups [37]. Latino American and Asian American are pan-ethnic terms, and researchers must consider the sociocultural diversity among Latino and Asian self- identified individuals. For example, the term Latino encompasses 28 different nationalities (e.g., Mexican, Ecuadorean, etc.). Similarly, the term Asian includes 32 different nationalities and ethnic groups (e.g., Chinese, Korean, etc.). Categorizing Latino American and Asian American as one racial group can overlook the diverse cultures of origins as well as diverse contexts (e.g., individuals in various sub-regions of the United States), which might be relevant to youth victimization and school bullying. Scholars need to consider identifying risk and protective factors for youth victimization and school bullying within Latino American and Asian American subgroups.

Regarding immigration, this book chapter focuses on youth victimization and school bullying research for the children of immigrants, defined as youth who are a part of an immigrant family or have at least one immigrant parent. We do not discuss, however, the importance of assimilation as related to youth victimization and school bullying. What is emerging from this research is a phenomenon called the "immigrant paradox," the counterintuitive finding that adapting or assimilating to U.S. cultural and social norms may result in adverse outcomes, such as youth victimization and school bullying. Studies reveal that for immigrants and their children, assimilation is associated with increased psychological and health problems, educational failure, and involvement in violence and victimization [11, 13, 37]. It is argued that the process of "becoming an American" is presumed to be one of becoming deviant and assimilating to the American phenomenon of a "moral rejection" of authority; thus, increasing contact with deviant youth increases involvement in deviance, aggressive, and potentially bullying behavior for the children of immigrants [11, 13, 37].

From a religious standpoint, Muslim Americans are not a monolithic group, nor can they be described exclusively in terms of a single common experience. Nonetheless, it is a term that millions of Muslims living in the United States use to identify themselves [15–17]. Muslim Americans come from at least 77 countries and include native-born Black/African Americans and other converts to Islam. Moreover, there is diversity concerning race, ethnicity, and immigrant experiences among Muslim Americans [15–17]. Similar to Latino Americans and Asian Americans, categorizing Muslim American youth monolithically can overlook their diverse cultures of origin, as well as diverse contexts (e.g., individuals in various sub-regions of the United States), which might be relevant to youth's experiences in victimization and school bullying. It is also evident that there is minimal research focusing on the victimization and school bullying experiences of Muslim American youth. As highlighted in the introductory chapter, the concept of intersectionality also matters when understanding how race, ethnicity, immigration, and religion are associated with school bullying. For instance, Asian American immigrant girls are significantly more susceptible to victimization at school, predominantly sexual harassment and violence [37].

Conclusion

Although we attempt to explicate how race, ethnicity, immigration, and religion are associated with school bullying, there is much more research needed to sufficiently understand and address bullying among racial, ethnic, immigrant, and religious minority youth whose experiences are embedded in the complex group, school, community, and social and cultural contexts across the United States. While we have examined emerging literature highlighting some of the ways these contexts impact the school experiences of these minority populations, we argue that additional research needs to investigate the risk and protective factors among these groups. Further, beyond additional efforts to identify these factors and their workings, we assert that the development of culturally appropriate intervention programs to strengthen and protect racial, ethnic, immigrant, and religious minorities in schools is a crucial next step in addressing this pervasive social problem. Finally, we would like to remind the reader that factors raised in this chapter about race, ethnicity, immigration, religion, and school bullying victimization can also intersect with socioeconomic and social status, family cohesion and interactions, sex, sexual orientation, gender identity, and gender expression, and disabilities and special health needs.

References

1. United States Census Bureau. (2014). *Current population survey*. Washington, DC: U.S.: Census Bureau, Population Division.
2. Musu-Gillette, L., Zhang, A., Wang, K., Zhang, J., & Oudekerk, B. (2017). *Indicators of school crime and safety: 2016 (NCES 2017–064/NCJ 250650)*. Washington, DC: National Center for Education Statistics, U.S. Department of Education, and Bureau of Justice Statistics, Office of Justice Programs, U.S. Department of Justice Programs, US Department of Justice.
3. Low, B. J., Fleschler, M., & Sinicrope, P. K. (2005). Prevalence of Hispanic child aggression and victimization. *Journal of Intercultural Disciplines, 5*, 75.
4. Mouttapa, M., Valente, T., Gallaher, P., Rohrbach, L. A., & Unger, J. B. (2004). Social network predictors of bullying and victimization. *Adolescence, 39*(154), 315.
5. Sawyer, A. L., Bradshaw, C. P., & O'Brennan, L. M. (2008). Examining ethnic, gender, and developmental differences in the way children report being a victim of "bullying" on self-report measures. *Journal of Adolescent Health, 43*(2), 106–114.
6. Williams, L. M., & Peguero, A. A. (2013). The impact of school bullying on racial/ethnic achievement. *Race and Social Problems, 5*(4), 296–308.
7. Goldweber, A., Waasdorp, T. E., & Bradshaw, C. P. (2013). Examining associations between race, urbanicity, and patterns of bullying involvement. *Journal of Youth and Adolescence, 42*(2), 206–219.
8. Hong, J. S., & Espelage, D. L. (2012). A review of research on bullying and peer victimization in school: An ecological system analysis. *Aggression and Violent Behavior, 17*(4), 311–322.
9. Kao, G., Vaquera, E., & Goyette, K. (2013). *Education and immigration*. John Wiley & Sons.
10. Suárez-Orozco, C., Suárez-Orozco, M., & Todorova, I. (2008). *Learning a new land: Educational pathways of immigrant youth*. Cambridge, MA: Harvard University Press.

11. Peguero, A. A. (2009). Victimizing the children of immigrants: Latino and Asian American student victimization. *Youth & Society, 41*(2), 186–208.
12. Peguero, A. A. (2012). Schools, bullying, and inequality: Intersecting factors and complexities with the stratification of youth victimization at school. *Sociology Compass, 6*(5), 402–412.
13. Peguero, A. A. (2013). An adolescent victimization immigrant paradox? School-based routines, lifestyles, and victimization across immigration generations. *Journal of Youth and Adolescence, 42*(11), 1759–1773.
14. Gonzales, R. G. (2015). *Lives in limbo: Undocumented and coming of age in America.* Berkeley, CA: University of California Press.
15. Abu El-Haj, T. R. (2007). "I was born here, but my home, it's not here": Educating for democratic citizenship in an era of transnational migration and global conflict. *Harvard Educational Review, 77*(3), 285–316.
16. Basford, L. (2010). From mainstream to east African charter: Cultural and religious experiences of Somali youth in US schools. *Journal of School Choice, 4*(4), 485–509.
17. Bonet, S. W. (2011). Educating Muslim American youth in a post-9/11 era: A critical review of policy and practice. *The High School Journal, 95*(1), 46–55.
18. Kozol, J. (2005). *The shame of the nation: The restoration of apartheid schooling in America.* Broadway Books.
19. Kozol, J. (2012). *Savage inequalities: Children in America's schools.* Broadway Books.
20. Lareau, A. (2011). *Unequal childhoods: Class, race, and family life.* University of California Press.
21. Lewis, A. E. (2003). *Race in the schoolyard: Reproducing the color line in school 2003b New Brunswick.* New Brunswick, NJ: Rutgers University Press.
22. Lewis, A. E., & Diamond, J. B. (2017). *Despite the best intentions: How racial inequality thrives in good schools.* Oxford University Press.
23. Hong, J. S., & Eamon, M. K. (2011). Students' perceptions of unsafe schools: An ecological systems analysis. *Journal of Child and Family Studies, 21*(3), 428–438.
24. Bradshaw, C. P., Waasdorp, T. E., Goldweber, A., & Johnson, S. L. (2013). Bullies, gangs, drugs, and school: Understanding the overlap and the role of ethnicity and urbanicity. *Journal of Youth and Adolescence, 42*(2), 220–234.
25. Rojas-Gaona, C. E., Hong, J. S., & Peguero, A. A. (2016). The significance of race/ethnicity in adolescent violence: A decade of review, 2005–2015. *Journal of Criminal Justice, 46*, 137–147.
26. Anderson, E. (1999). *Code of the street: Decency, violence, and the moral life of the inner city.* New York: Norton.
27. Rios, V. M. (2011). *Punished: Policing the lives of Black and Latino boys.* NYU Press.
28. Rios, V. M. (2017). *Human targets: Schools, police, and the criminalization of Latino youth.* University of Chicago Press.
29. Brunson, R. K., & Miller, J. (2009). Schools, neighborhoods, and adolescent conflicts: A situational examination of reciprocal dynamics. *Justice Quarterly, 26*(2), 183–210.
30. Peguero, A. A., Popp, A. M., Latimore, T. L., Shekarkhar, Z., & Koo, D. J. (2011). Social control theory and school misbehavior: Examining the role of race and ethnicity. *Youth Violence and Juvenile Justice, 9*(3), 259–275.
31. Sykes, B. L., Piquero, A. R., & Gioviano, J. P. (2017). Code of the classroom? Social disadvantage and bullying among American adolescents, US 2011-2012. *Crime & Delinquency, 63*(14), 1883–1922.
32. Renzulli, L. A., & Evans, L. (2005). School choice, charter schools, and white flight. *Social Problems, 52*(3), 398–418.
33. Welch, K., & Payne, A. A. (2012). Exclusionary school punishment: The effect of racial threat on expulsion and suspension. *Youth Violence and Juvenile Justice, 10*(2), 155–171.
34. Peguero, A. A., & Bondy, J. M. (2015). Schools, justice, and immigrant students: Segmented assimilation, race, ethnicity, gender, and perceptions of fairness and order. *Teachers College Record, 117*(7), n7.

35. Peguero, A. A., & Bondy, J. M. (2020). The importance of immigration with future research about school safety. *Race and Justice, 10*(3), 247–268.
36. Portes, A., & Rumbaut, R. G. (2014). *Immigrant America: A portrait*. University of California Press.
37. Hong, J. S., Peguero, A. A., Choi, S., Lanesskog, D., Espelage, D. L., & Lee, N. Y. (2014). Social ecology of bullying and peer victimization of Latino and Asian youth in the United States: A review of the literature. *Journal of School Violence, 13*(3), 315–338.
38. Peguero, A. A., & Williams, L. M. (2013). Racial and ethnic stereotypes and bullying victimization. *Youth & Society, 45*(4), 545–564.
39. Phelan, J. E., & Rudman, L. A. (2010). Reactions to ethnic deviance: The role of backlash in racial stereotype maintenance. *Journal of Personality and Social Psychology, 99*(2), 265.
40. Fordham, S., & Ogbu, J. U. (1986). Black students' school success: Coping with the "burden of 'acting white'". *The Urban Review, 18*(3), 176–206.
41. Wilcox, P., Tillyer, M. S., & Fisher, B. S. (2009). Gendered opportunity? School-based adolescent victimization. *Journal of Research in Crime and Delinquency, 46*(2), 245–269.
42. Peguero, A. A., Popp, A. M., & Koo, D. J. (2015). Race, ethnicity, and school-based adolescent victimization. *Crime & Delinquency, 61*(3), 323–349.

Chapter 7
Bullying and Youth with Disabilities and Special Health Needs: Victimizing Students with Physical, Emotional/Behavioral, and Learning Disorders

Abstract In Chap. 7, we discuss how and why youth with disabilities and special health needs are vulnerable to bullying at school. Research suggests that youth with learning and developmental disabilities are at an elevated risk of peer victimization. Youth with observable disabilities in segregated settings are more likely to be victimized by their peers without disabilities in school than those with non-observable disabilities. Psychosocial problems, such as depression and anxiety, are also factors related to the likelihood of being bullied at school. Depressed youth are more likely to be victimized by their peers than are children without a history of depression.

Keywords Physical disabilities · Emotional/behavioral disorders · Learning disorders

Introduction

In recent years, several incidences of bullying involving students with disabilities have headline news. For instance, in May of 2014, Burris Hurd, a father of a 9-year-old boy with autism in Richmond, California, boarded a school bus and attacked the student who allegedly bullied his son. Hurd grabbed the 11-year-old bully by the hair, pulled the boy out of his seat, and shoved him into the side of the bus. Hurd was charged with child abuse and corporal injury to a child [1]. Children with disabilities tend to be overprotected by their parents as, according to the United Nations Children's Fund [2], they "are one of the most marginalized and excluded groups in society." They encounter discrimination in various forms, from negative attitudes to being excluded from rights to healthcare, education, and survival. Disabilities can begin anytime during the developmental period and can last throughout an individual's lifetime [3]. The Centers for Disease Control and Prevention reports that in the United States, about one in six, or 15% of children ages 3 through 17 have one or more developmental disabilities, including attention-deficit/hyperactivity disorder,

A. A. Peguero, J. S. Hong, *School Bullying*, Springer Series on Child and Family Studies, https://doi.org/10.1007/978-3-030-64367-6_7

autism spectrum disorder, cerebral palsy, hearing loss, intellectual disability, learning disability, vision impairment, and other types of developmental delays [4]. Because children and adolescents with disabilities may be perceived to be "different," they may be at a higher risk of being bullied in their school relative to their peers without any disabilities. These children are particularly vulnerable because their disability can make it difficult to identify the types of bullying that are happening.

In this chapter, we examine bullying and peer victimization involving children and adolescents with three types of disabilities—physical disabilities, emotional/behavioral disorders, and learning disorders. We first discuss the types of developmental disabilities and how they may relate to bullying and peer victimization. We then present multiple level factors associated with bullying and peer victimization in children with disabilities within the social-ecological context. In the final section of this chapter, we highlight the complexities associated with developmental disabilities and bullying and victimization.

Physical Disabilities

A *physical disability* is defined as any intrinsic biological or acquired condition that permanently prevents normal body movement [5], causes impairments, and consequently interferes with the development or function of the central nervous system, muscles, joints, and/or bones. Children with a physical disability may have impairments such as cerebral palsy, spina bifida, muscular dystrophy, arthritis, developmental coordination disorder, amputations, genetic disorders, and so forth. According to a study conducted by the American Academy of Pediatrics [6], the prevalence of childhood physical disability increased by 16.3% between 2001–2002 and 2010–2011. Children with a physical disability have special health needs (e.g., epilepsy or food allergen) which place them at an increased risk of bully victimization because of physical vulnerabilities, social skill challenges, and intolerant social environment [7]. Several studies have reported a significantly higher prevalence of bully victimization experienced by children with physical-type of disabilities compared to those with typical development. For instance, one study, which conducted separate, in-depth interviews with 13-year-olds diagnosed with an autism spectrum disorder, intellectual disability, or typical development, found that children with autism spectrum disorder were more frequently victimized than those with an intellectual disability and those with typical development [8]. Another study, which compared the prevalence and intensity of victimization of adolescents with chronic conditions (defined as those with chronic disease and/or physical disability) to those without any chronic conditions, also found that those with chronic conditions were victims of two or three forms of bullying [9]. These adolescents were also more likely than non-victims to be depressed, to have physical symptoms, be in a poorer school climate, and have been victims of violence [9]. More recently, a limited number of studies have been conducted on experiences in bullying among children with food allergies [10, 11]. Lieberman et al. [10] found that of the respondents with food allergies, 24% reported that they had been bullied, harassed, and teased because of their food allergies. Similar to Lieberman et al.'s (2010) study, Shemesh et al. [11] found that 24.7% of parents with children reported that their child was bullied specifically due to food allergy, which was also associated with lower quality of life and increased distress. Muraro et al. [12], on the other hand, found a much higher prevalence of bullying victimization among allergic patients. The study findings revealed that 60% of food-allergic children reported being victims of bullying at least once within the last 2 months. Also, the probability of bullying victimization was found to be twice higher among food-allergic children than among non-allergic children [12].

Emotional/Behavioral Disorders

Children with emotional and behavioral problems frequently experience distress and can suffer substantially as they may demonstrate impairments across multiple domains, such as problematic interactions with peers, dysfunctional parent-child relationships, lack of physical safety, inability to participate in childcare, school problems, and physical health problems [13]. Well-developed literature over the years have reported emotional and behavioral outcomes of bullying and peer victimization [e.g., 14–16]. Similarly, youth with emotional and behavioral disorders are at a heightened risk of bullying, as indicated in a study by Coolidge, DenBoer, and Segal [17], which found that bullying behavior was correlated with Axis II diagnoses of passive-aggressive, histrionic, paranoid, and dependent disorder. Other studies also found that symptoms of behavioral disorders, including conduct disorder, oppositional defiant disorder, ADHD, and low self-esteem were predictive of bullying and peer victimization [18–23]. Children considered anxious-withdrawn or described as having a personality disorder may exhibit low self-esteem and maybe shy and suffer from unhappiness [24], making them possible targets for bullies. Further, from a study using a nationally representative survey of students with disabilities, Blake, Lund, Zhou, Kwok, and Benz [25] reported that the rate of bullying victimization was among the highest for students with emotional problems.

Recent studies have also identified specific forms of behavioral disorders, particularly autism spectrum disorder (ASD) as significant predictors of bullying and peer victimization [8, 26–28]. In terms of ASD, youth with ASD are more likely to be victimized in school relative to their peers without ASD [26, 27]. For example, one study using a nationally representative sample [27] found that the prevalence rate of bullying involvement for youth with an ASD were 46.3% for victimization, 14.8% for perpetration, and 8.9% for victimization/perpetration. Another study also reported that the prevalence rate of bullying and peer victimization between 6% and 46% [28]. Also, youth with ASD reported being victimized more frequently than their peers with an intellectual disability or of typical development, and these youth were more likely to experience different types of bullying relative to their peers [8].

Learning Disorders

It is not unusual for children to have trouble with reading, writing, or other learning-related tasks at some point in their life. However, according to the Learning Disabilities Association of America [29] children with learning disabilities commonly exhibit symptoms including short attention span, poor memory, difficulty following directions; inability to discriminate between or among letters; numbers or signs; poor reading and/or writing ability; problems with eye-hand coordination; difficulties with sequencing; and disorganization. Although these symptoms can be found in all children at some point in their life, children with learning disabilities have a cluster of these symptoms that do not disappear [29]. Similar to physical disabilities and emotional and behavioral disorders, adolescents who are diagnosed with a learning disorder have a significantly higher risk of bullying than those without learning disorders [30, 31]. According to a study conducted by Little [31], the prevalence rate of bullying victimization in children with Asperger's and non-verbal learning disorder was 94%; of these, mothers of these reported that almost three-quarters of their children had been physically victimized by their peers or sibling; and 75% had been emotionally bullied. Rose, Espelage, and Monda-Amaya's [32] study findings from a large sample of middle and high school students also suggest that adolescents in a special education program reported greater rates of bullying, fighting, and victimization than students in the general education. Another study by Reiter and Lapidot-Lefler [33], which included a sample of 186 students with intellectual disabilities, found that those who identified as bullies and bully/victims tended to exhibit significantly high levels of a temper tantrum, unruly and quarrelsome behavior, and a tendency to lie and steal. The study also found that those who were victimized displayed emotional and interpersonal problems [33]. Similar to other studies, Swearer, Wang, Maag, Siebecker, and Frerichs' [34] study suggests that students with behavioral disorders and those with observable disabilities in special education reported being victimized more than those in the general education pool.

However, a review of bullying involvement of children in special education also found that although students with learning disabilities are victimized more frequently than those without disabilities, findings related to the prevalence and predictors have been inconsistent [35]. One study found that between 4% and 9% of students with intellectual and developmental disabilities reported bullying or victimization at least once a week [36]. It is also interesting to note that although the rate of victimization is higher among students with a disability, those with a higher incidence of learning disabilities experience less victimization than those with more severe cognitive or physical disabilities [35]. Still, youth with a learning disorder seem to be at risk of peer victimization and peer rejection at the hands of their peers, as they may display problematic characteristics, behaviors, and psychosocial problems that resemble other groups of children who are frequently bullied in school [37].

Social-Ecological Framework

The social-ecological framework, an extension of Bronfenbrenner's [38] ecological model of child development, posits that interactions among individual, peer group, institutional, community, and societal factors influence or inhibit adolescent behaviors and attitudes. It is important to examine bullying participation [39] of children and adolescents with disabilities, taking into account the social-ecological framework [32]. In this section, bullying and peer victimization experiences of children and adolescents with disabilities within the societal, community, institutional, peer group, and individual contexts will be explored.

Societal

The societal level consists of broad level factors that create a climate in which bullying may be encouraged or discouraged. One example would be laws, or the lack thereof. Although federal law does not directly address bullying, federally-funded schools are mandated to resolve bullying and harassment. Schools receiving federal funding are required by federal laws to address conduct that creates a hostile school environment, which would interfere with students' ability to participate in or benefit from the school [7]. The federal laws enforced by the U.S. Department of Education and the U.S. Department of Justice require schools to address bullying and harassment based on the student's race, color, national origin, sex, religion, or disabilities [7]. More specifically, federal civil rights laws passed by the U.S. Department of Education and the Department of Justice mandate that failure to respond appropriately to bullying and harassment of students based on a protected class (which includes disability status) is a violation of one or more civil rights following the *Title IV and Title VI of the Civil Rights Act* (1964), *Title IX of the Education Amendments* (1972), *Section 504 of the Rehabilitation Act* (1973), *Title II and III of the Americans with Disabilities Act*, and the *Individuals with Disabilities Education Act* [7]. Bullying behavior can be regarded as "disability harassment," which is prohibited under Section. 504 of the *Rehabilitation Act of 1973* and Title II of the *Americans with Disabilities Act of 1990*. A "disability harassment" is referred to as "intimidation or abusive behavior toward a student based on a disability that creates a hostile [school] environment by interfering with or denying a student's participation in or receipt of benefits, services, or opportunities in the institution's program" [40]. Under Section 504 and Title II, a school's inappropriate or lacking response to the harassment of students with disabilities would constitute disability harassment, and schools that fail to protect students with disabilities from harassment can face a lawsuit [41]. In 2012, the Second Circuit Court upheld a million-dollar verdict against a school district in New York, which was sued by a student who had endured over 3 years of harassment. Although the school did everything required in most anti-bullying statutes, such as implementing a policy against bullying, having a reporting system, and holding training, the school ignored many signs that more action was needed to address the "culture of bias," which reinforced disability harassment in school [41].

Community

Settings such as schools and homes are a part of the community where social relationships and peer interactions occur. Children and adolescents spend the majority of their days within school systems where bullying and peer victimization most frequently occur in the school setting. Most school districts in the U.S. have been structured to divide students into groups, which emphasizes differences rather than commonalities. This is particularly apparent in the design of special education programs. However, for students with disabilities, their "odd" or "inappropriate" behaviors may play a role in attracting bullies in an integrated environment (e.g., classroom) where students with disabilities frequently occupy the bottom rung of the student hierarchy [42]. According to one study finding [43], children who are diagnosed with Asperger's disorder and attending a public school or a school with a general education student population were at the highest risk of being victimized. Moreover, the study found that those in full inclusion classrooms were more likely to be victimized than those who spent the majority of their time in special education settings [43]. Not surprisingly, a significant proportion of adolescents with learning difficulties report that they prefer learning in a special education setting as opposed to a mainstream classroom setting, although students in special education settings experienced far more bullying than those in a specialized classroom setting [44]. More broadly, bullying and harassment of students with disabilities in inclusive classrooms can be influenced by community perceptions and views on disability. As stated by Baker and Donelly [45], addressing and preventing bullying of students with disabilities is limited "if the community view [sic] disability negatively, if the family is not supported to provide social opportunities, and if the school cannot provide the environment in which to learn new social skills" [p. 82]. Researchers have recommended that it is important to recognize that school climate and community attitudes that are tolerant of bullying and promote negative attitudes toward students with disabilities need to change [37]. Furthermore, several scholars have also suggested that more systemic interventions are needed, such as changing the school and community to assist children with disabilities with inclusion by peers [37, 46, 47].

Institutional

To date, the literature on the relevance of institutional settings in bullying of youth with disabilities is absent, although a limited number of studies have explored institutional factors associated with bullying in the workplace and military settings. *Institutions* can be conceived of as the structural manifestation of social norms [48]. Extant research suggests that characteristics of institutional settings (notably, schools and workplaces), such as attitudes supportive of aggression and violence, can increase the likelihood of bullying, targeting those who are perceived as weak and vulnerable, such as students with disabilities. According to Unnever and Cornell [49], which examined the nature and extent of students' attitudes toward bullying in six middle schools, a culture of bullying is pervasive among middle school students and those with pro-bullying attitudes are more likely to engage in such behavior. The pervasive culture of bullying, combined with adverse outcomes of school climates that are supportive of aggression and dominance (e.g., suicide), have highlighted a renewed desire for school officials to address ways of eliminating the culture of bullying and harassment which are prevalent in public schools, especially a culture that condones targeting students for their differences [50]. In South Carolina, legislators responded to the culture of bullying in June of 2006 with the passage of the *Safe School Climate Act*, which was designed to address how the school, as an institution, handled bullying situations [50]. The Act also required school districts in South Carolina to establish policies to address the culture of bullying before January 1, 2007. However, as indicated in Terry's [50] study findings, bullying is a complex phenomenon and the culture of bullying continues to be the subject of debate among researchers, school psychologists, and other relevant stakeholders. In addition to tackling the culture of bullying, a limited number of scholars have also proposed that effectively preventing bullying necessitates institutional support in the form of teacher support and a cultural shift that supports the process of bullying prevention [e.g., 51, 52].

Peer

Children's and adolescents' peer group support, or peer support, has been recognized as a salient protective factor that can reduce the probability of peer victimization and the adverse outcomes of being peers victimized, such as psychological distress and low life satisfaction [53, 54]. It has been well established in the research literature that children's mental health can be severely undermined by frequent bullying experiences at school, which can also be exacerbated by having inadequate social support, particularly from their peers [54]. Further, given that students adopt a variety of coping strategies when they experience peer victimization, the likelihood of seeking help when bullied will depend on the school context [55]; one important component of school context is the existence of a peer support system [55]. As such, there has been growing interest in elevating peer support as an approach to bullying prevention in various countries, including Canada, Australia, and New Zealand. As empirical literature demonstrates, increased peer support was found to be the most significant predictor of decreased victimization, particularly for students with disabilities [e.g., 32, 56]. One study, which examined the bullying experiences of students diagnosed with autism spectrum disorders, found that these students received lower levels of social support from parents, classmates, and teachers than students in the general education pool, as well as those with dyslexia [56]. However, social support from classmates was found to be the most significant predictor in a reduced frequency of bullying [56]. However, as Cowie [57] had argued, the dynamics of adolescent peer relations are very complex, and it is insufficient to simply adopt a peer support strategy to avoid bullying. Because many children and adolescents tend to look down on victims of bullying, asking peer groups for help may not always be an effective strategy [58]. Also, children with disabilities are less likely to report or seek peer support than those without disabilities [59, 60] for social desirability reasons [59]. Early identification of negative peer interactions, in conjunction with an intervention that facilitates positive peer interactions, can ensure that negative behavior patterns among youth do not become entrenched [61].

Individual

Individual characteristics and personal attributes, such as the nature and severity of the disabilities, are identified as a factor in peer victimization of youth with disabilities. For example, students with cognitive disabilities [33] and those with language problems reported being victimized more frequently compared to their peers in general educational settings [62, 63]. Moreover, certain individual characteristics can heighten risks for being a victim of bullying among youth with disabilities, such as problem behavior and poor social skills [see 35, for a review]. A recent review of the literature on bullying experiences of students with ASD also suggests that characteristics at the individual level, such as social vulnerability, behavioral problems, racial identity, academic performance, and age were significant correlates [64]. Research has also identified other psychosocial characteristics of children with disabilities that can elevate their risk of peer victimization, including symptoms of withdrawal behavior, anxiety, depressive symptoms, thought problems, attention problems [65], and anger [66]. Fewer studies have identified promotive factors at the individual level concerning peer victimization risk involving youth with disabilities. One study [30] did find that secure parental attachment [30] was negatively associated with peer victimization risks among children with disabilities.

Complexities

Although emerging bodies of research literature have explored the significance of bullying and peer victimization involving students with disabilities, several complexities need to be considered. In terms of the types of disabilities, students with physical disabilities, emotional and behavioral disorders, and learning disorders are significantly at risk of being victimized in school due to perceived differences. However, it is also important to mention that bullying of children with disabilities is complex, and as a limited number of studies suggest, students with emotional or learning disorders might be at a significantly higher risk of victimization by their peers, relative to youth with physical disabilities. It is unclear why students with emotional or learning disorders are more at risk of being bullied than those with physical disabilities. Conceivably, certain students, such as those in a wheelchair or those with visual impairment, may be less likely to be physically assaulted because they are perceived as being "fragile," although they might be teased and taunted by their peers. Additional research might qualitatively explore whether there are any differences in peer dynamics and bullying experiences among adolescents of various types of disabilities.

It is also important that although the rate of bullying involvement is higher among these adolescents, there is a need to explore whether bullying is higher among these populations when intersecting with other social identities. Is bullying higher among adolescents with a learning disorder who may also belong to a racial and ethnic minority group? Adolescents who are a racial and ethnic minority, particularly African Americans with ADHD are less likely to show lower treatment rates due to lack of culturally viable assessment tools and access to treatment [see [67]], placing them even at a higher risk of bullying involvement. Oftentimes, due to language barriers, racial and ethnic minorities such as immigrant youth are often perceived as having a learning disorder or placed in a special education program, which can exacerbate their likelihood of being confronted with peer victimization.

Regarding the social-ecological framework, which identified factors associated with bullying and victimization at the societal, community, institutional, peer, and individual contexts, a large body of research has assessed, for example, school and peer-level factors. However, although the federal laws have been enacted to address bullying and harassment of students who belong to a protected class, such as those with disabilities [7], research to date has not empirically examined whether such policies have been effective in reducing the risk of peer victimization of students with disabilities and those in a special education program. However, since 2009, the Department of Education's Office of Civil Rights stated that it had received more than 2000 complaints related to bullying of adolescents with disabilities [68]. Likewise, although institutional factors, such as a culture of bullying and pro-violence attitude in the school settings are found to be positively linked to an adolescent's risk of bullying [49], it is unclear whether a culture of bullying can also increase bullying risks among students with disabilities. Furthermore, as previously mentioned, while a great deal of empirical investigation on the risk factors at the individual level associated with peer victimization exists, there is a limited number of studies considering protective factors. For example, despite their perceived differences, students with disabilities, particularly those with physical forms of disability, may be supported by their teachers in school. These youth are also more likely to have parents who are involved in their school activities, which can shield them from victimization.

Conclusion

It has been well established that bullying in school has a significant impact on the learning environment and on the mental health of the youth involved, which can be a detriment to themselves, to the school environment, and the society at large. For several years, school districts have expended a considerable amount of their energy and their resources to manage problem behavior, promote the development of prosocial behavior, and expand mental health services for children in school. Considering that school bullying is significantly higher among students with disabilities, we have attempted to provide an overview of how disability status and special education are linked to school bullying. Beyond additional efforts to identify factors associated with bullying and peer victimization, we assert that anti-bullying interventions that are specific to the needs of students with disabilities are an important next step for the development of accessible and inclusive education, as these students have long been denied equal opportunities to maximize their learning potential.

References

1. Thompson, V. (2014). Bullying of students with disabilities in our schools. *SWHELPER*. Retrieved August 18, 2020, from https://swhelper.org/2014/06/26/bullying-students-disabilities-schools/
2. UNICEF. (n.d.). *Disabilities*. UNICEF. Retrieved August 18, 2020, from https://www.unicef.org/disabilities/.
3. Centers for Disease Control and Prevention. (2018). *Facts about developmental disabilities*. Centers for Disease Control and Prevention. Retrieved August 18, 2020, from https://www.cdc.gov/ncbddd/developmentaldisabilities/facts.html.
4. Boyle, C. A., Boulet, S., Schieve, L. A., Cohen, R. A., Blumberg, S. J., Yeargin-Allsopp, M., Kogan, M. D., et al. (2011). Trends in the prevalence of developmental disabilities in US children, 1997–2008. *Pediatrics, 127*(6), 1034–1042.
5. Child and Youth Health. (2017). Physical disability—children. *Child and Youth Health*. Retrieved from http://www.cyh.com/HealthTopics/HealthTopicDetails.aspx?p=114&np=306&id=1874
6. American Academy of Pediatrics. (2013). Childhood disability rate jumps 16 percent over past decade. *ScienceDaily*. Retrieved August 18, 2020, from https://www.sciencedaily.com/releases/2013/05/130505073733.htm.
7. Stopbullying.gov. (2019). Federal Laws. *StopBullying.gov*. Text. Retrieved August 18, 2020, from https://www.stopbullying.gov/resources/laws/federal

8. Zeedyk, S., Rodriguez, G., Tipton, L., Baker, B., & Blacher, J. (2014). Bullying of youth with autism spectrum disorder, intellectual disability, or typical development: Victim and parent perspectives. *Research in Autism Spectrum Disorders, 8*(9), 1173–1183.
9. Pittet, I., Berchtold, A., Akré, C., Michaud, P.-A., & Suris, J.-C. (2010). Are adolescents with chronic conditions particularly at risk for bullying? *Archives of Disease in Childhood, 95*(9), 711–716.
10. Lieberman, J. A., Weiss, C., Furlong, T. J., Sicherer, M., & Sicherer, S. H. (2010). Bullying among pediatric patients with food allergy. *Annals of Allergy, Asthma & Immunology, 105*(4), 282–286.
11. Shemesh, E., Annunziato, R. A., Ambrose, M. A., Ravid, N. L., Mullarkey, C., Rubes, M., Sicherer, S. H., et al. (2013). Child and parental reports of bullying in a consecutive sample of children with food allergy. *Pediatrics, 131*(1), e10–e17.
12. Muraro, A., Polloni, L., Lazzarotto, F., Toniolo, A., Baldi, I., Bonaguro, R., Masiello, M., et al. (2014). Comparison of bullying of food-allergic versus healthy schoolchildren in Italy. *Journal of Allergy and Clinical Immunology, 134*(3), 749–751.
13. Gleason, M. M., Goldson, E., Yogman, M. W., Child, C., on P. A. of Health F, et al. (2016). Addressing early childhood emotional and behavioral problems. *Pediatrics, 138*(6), e20163025.
14. Bond, L., Carlin, J. B., Thomas, L., Rubin, K., & Patton, G. (2001). Does bullying cause emotional problems? A prospective study of young teenagers. *BMJ, 323*(7311), 480–484.
15. Copeland, W. E., Wolke, D., Angold, A., & Costello, E. J. (2013). Adult psychiatric outcomes of bullying and being bullied by peers in childhood and adolescence. *JAMA Psychiatry, 70*(4), 419–426.
16. Gini, G. (2008). Associations between bullying behaviour, psychosomatic complaints, emotional and behavioural problems. *Journal of Paediatrics and Child Health, 44*(9), 492–497.
17. Coolidge, F. L., DenBoer, J. W., & Segal, D. L. (2004). Personality and neuropsychological correlates of bullying behavior. *Personality and Individual Differences, 36*(7), 1559–1569.
18. Holmberg, K., & Hjern, A. (2008). Bullying and attention-deficit–hyperactivity disorder in 10-year-olds in a Swedish community. *Developmental Medicine & Child Neurology, 50*(2), 134–138.
19. Kokkinos, C. M., & Panayiotou, G. (2004). Predicting bullying and victimization among early adolescents: Associations with disruptive behavior disorders. *Aggressive Behavior, 30*(6), 520–533.
20. Kowalski, R. M., & Fedina, C. (2011). Cyber bullying in ADHD and Asperger syndrome populations. *Research in Autism Spectrum Disorders, 5*(3), 1201–1208.
21. Sciberras, E., Ohan, J., & Anderson, V. (2012). Bullying and peer victimisation in adolescent girls with attention-deficit/hyperactivity disorder. *Child Psychiatry & Human Development, 43*(2), 254–270.
22. Turner, H. A., Vanderminden, J., Finkelhor, D., Hamby, S., & Shattuck, A. (2011). Disability and victimization in a national sample of children and youth. *Child Maltreatment, 16*(4), 275–286.
23. Zablotsky, B., Bradshaw, C. P., Anderson, C., & Law, P. A. (2013). The association between bullying and the psychological functioning of children with autism spectrum disorders. *Journal of Developmental & Behavioral Pediatrics, 34*(1), 1–8.
24. Heward, W. L. (2003). *Exceptional children: An introduction to special education*. Merrill/Prentice Hall.
25. Blake, J. J., Lund, E. M., Zhou, Q., Kwok, O., & Benz, M. R. (2012). National prevalence rates of bully victimization among students with disabilities in the United States. *School Psychology Quarterly, 27*(4), 210.
26. Kloosterman, P. H., Kelley, E. A., Craig, W. M., Parker, J. D., & Javier, C. (2013). Types and experiences of bullying in adolescents with an autism spectrum disorder. *Research in Autism Spectrum Disorders, 7*(7), 824–832.

27. Sterzing, P. R., Shattuck, P. T., Narendorf, S. C., Wagner, M., & Cooper, B. P. (2012). Prevalence and correlates of bullying involvement among adolescents with an autism Spectrum disorder. *Archives of Pediatrics & Adolescent Medicine, 166*(11), 1058.
28. Van Roekel, E., Scholte, R. H., & Didden, R. (2010). Bullying among adolescents with autism spectrum disorders: Prevalence and perception. *Journal of Autism and Developmental Disorders, 40*(1), 63–73.
29. Learning Disabilities Association of America. (n.d.). Symptoms of learning disabilities—Learning Disabilities Association of America. *Symptoms of learning disabilities*. Retrieved August 18, 2020, from https://ldaamerica.org/info/symptoms-of-learning-disabilities/
30. Klomek, A. B., Kopelman-Rubin, D., Al-Yagon, M., Berkowitz, R., Apter, A., & Mikulincer, M. (2016). Victimization by bullying and attachment to parents and teachers among students who report learning disorders and/or attention deficit hyperactivity disorder. *Learning Disability Quarterly, 39*(3), 182–190.
31. Little, L. (2002). Middle-class mothers' perceptions of peer and sibling victimization among children with Asperger's syndrome and nonverbal learning disorders. *Issues in Comprehensive Pediatric Nursing, 25*(1), 43–57.
32. Rose, C. A., Espelage, D. L., Monda-Amaya, L. E., Shogren, K. A., & Aragon, S. R. (2015). Bullying and middle school students with and without specific learning disabilities: An examination of social-ecological predictors. *Journal of Learning Disabilities, 48*(3), 239–254.
33. Reiter, S., & Lapidot-Lefler, N. (2007). Bullying among special education students with intellectual disabilities: Differences in social adjustment and social skills. *Intellectual and Developmental Disabilities, 45*(3), 174–181.
34. Swearer, S. M., Wang, C., Maag, J. W., Siebecker, A. B., & Frerichs, L. J. (2012). Understanding the bullying dynamic among students in special and general education. *Journal of School Psychology, 50*(4), 503–520.
35. Rose, C. A., Monda-Amaya, L. E., & Espelage, D. L. (2011). Bullying perpetration and victimization in special education: A review of the literature. *Remedial and Special Education, 32*(2), 114–130.
36. Didden, R., Scholte, R. H., Korzilius, H., De Moor, J. M., Vermeulen, A., O'Reilly, M., Lancioni, G. E., et al. (2009). Cyberbullying among students with intellectual and developmental disability in special education settings. *Developmental Neurorehabilitation, 12*(3), 146–151.
37. Mishna, F. (2003). Learning disabilities and bullying: Double jeopardy. *Journal of Learning Disabilities, 36*(4), 336–347.
38. Bronfenbrenner, U. (1986). Ecology of the family as a context for human development: Research perspectives. *Developmental Psychology, 22*(6), 723.
39. Dempsey, J. P., Fireman, G. D., & Wang, E. (2006). Transitioning out of peer victimization in school children: Gender and behavioral characteristics. *Journal of Psychopathology and Behavioral Assessment, 28*(4), 271–280.
40. U.S. Department of Education. (2000). Prohibited disability harassment: Reminder of responsibilities under Section 504 of the Rehabilitation Act of 1973 and Title II of the Americans with Disabilities Act. *U.S. Department of Education*. Retrieved from www.ed.gov/about/offices/list/ocr/docs/disabharassltr.html
41. The Social Express. (2015). Bullying, students with disabilities, and social emotional skills. *The Social Express*. Retrieved August 18, 2020, from http://thesocialexpress.com/bullying-students-with-disabilities-and-social-emotional-skills/.
42. Hoover, J., & Stenhjem, P. (2003). Bullying and teasing of youth with disabilities: Creating positive school environments for effective inclusion. *Issue Brief, 2*(3) National Center on Secondary Education and Transition (NCSET), University of Minnesota.
43. Zablotsky, B., Bradshaw, C. P., Anderson, C. M., & Law, P. (2014). Risk factors for bullying among children with autism spectrum disorders. *Autism, 18*(4), 419–427.
44. Norwich, B., & Kelly, N. (2004). Pupils' views on inclusion: Moderate learning difficulties and bullying in mainstream and special schools. *British Educational Research Journal, 30*(1), 43–65.

45. Baker, K., & Donelly, M. (2001). The social experiences of children with disability and the influence of environment: A framework for intervention. *Disability & Society, 16*(1), 71–85.
46. Lewandowski, L. J., & Barlow, J. R. (2000). Social cognition and verbal learning disabilities. *Journal of Psychotherapy in Independent Practice, 1*(4), 35–47.
47. Pearl, R., & Bay, M. (1999). Psychosocial correlates of learning disabilities. In *Handbook of psychosocial characteristics of exceptional children* (pp. 443–470). Springer.
48. DeJordy, R., & Barrett, F. (2014). Emotions in institutions: Bullying as a mechanism of institutional control. In N. M. Ashkanasy, W. J. Zerbe, & C. E. J. Hatel (Eds.), *Emotions and the organizational fabric (research on emotion in organizations, Vol. 10)* (pp. 219–243). Emerald Group Publishing Limited.
49. Unnever, J. D., & Cornell, D. G. (2003). The culture of bullying in middle school. *Journal of School Violence, 2*(2), 5–27.
50. Terry, T. M. (2010). Blocking the bullies: Has South Carolina's safe school climate act made public schools safer? *The Clearinghouse, 83*(3), 96–100.
51. Glasner, A. T. (2010). On the front lines: Educating teachers about bullying and prevention methods. *Journal of Social Sciences, 6*, 537–541.
52. Ritchie, J., & O'Connell, T. (2001). Restorative justice and the contest between the relational and institutional paradigms. In J. Braithwaite & H. Strang (Eds.), *Restorative justice and civil society* (pp. 149–164). Cambridge, MA: Cambridge University Press.
53. Flaspohler, P. D., Elfstrom, J. L., Vanderzee, K. L., Sink, H. E., & Birchmeier, Z. (2009). Stand by me: The effects of peer and teacher support in mitigating the impact of bullying on quality of life. *Psychology in the Schools, 46*(7), 636–649.
54. Rigby, K. (2000). Effects of peer victimization in schools and perceived social support on adolescent Well-being. *Journal of Adolescence, 23*(1), 57–68.
55. Smith, P. K. (2004). Bullying: Recent developments. *Child and Adolescent Mental Health, 9*(3), 98–103.
56. Humphrey, N., & Symes, W. (2010). Perceptions of social support and experience of bullying among pupils with autistic spectrum disorders in mainstream secondary schools. *European Journal of Special Needs Education, 25*(1), 77–91.
57. Cowie, H. (2000). Bystanding or standing by: Gender issues in coping with bullying in English schools. *Aggressive Behavior, 26*(1), 85–97.
58. Cowie, H. (2011). Peer support as an intervention to counteract school bullying: Listen to the children. *Children & Society, 25*(4), 287–292.
59. Pellegrini, A. D. (2001). Sampling instances of victimization in middle school. In J. Juvonen & S. Graham (Eds.), *Peer harassment in school: The plight of the vulnerable and victimized* (pp. 125–146). New York, NY: Guilford.
60. Wenz-Gross, M., & Siperstein, G. N. (1997). Importance of social support in the adjustment of children with learning problems. *Exceptional Children, 63*(2), 183–193.
61. Cappadocia, M. C., Weiss, J. A., & Pepler, D. (2012). Bullying experiences among children and youth with autism spectrum disorders. *Journal of Autism and Developmental Disorders, 42*(2), 266–277.
62. Davis, S., Howell, P., & Cooke, F. (2002). Sociodynamic relationships between children who stutter and their non-stuttering classmates. *Journal of Child Psychology and Psychiatry, 43*(7), 939–947.
63. Knox, E., & Conti-Ramsden, G. (2003). Bullying risks of 11-year-old children with specific language impairment (SLI): Does school placement matter? *International Journal of Language & Communication Disorders, 38*(1), 1–12.
64. Sreckovic, M. A., Brunsting, N. C., & Able, H. (2014). Victimization of students with autism spectrum disorder: A review of prevalence and risk factors. *Research in Autism Spectrum Disorders, 8*(9), 1155–1172.
65. Baumeister, A. L., Storch, E. A., & Geffken, G. R. (2008). Peer victimization in children with learning disabilities. *Child and Adolescent Social Work Journal, 25*(1), 11–23.

66. Rose, C. A., & Espelage, D. L. (2012). Risk and protective factors associated with the bullying involvement of students with emotional and behavioral disorders. *Behavioral Disorders, 37*(3), 133–148.
67. Miller, T. W., Nigg, J. T., & Miller, R. L. (2009). Attention deficit hyperactivity disorder in African American children: What can be concluded from the past ten years? *Clinical Psychology Review, 29*(1), 77–86.
68. Diament, M. (2014). Feds warn schools on bullying of kids with disabilities. *Disability Scoop*. Retrieved August 18, 2020, from https://www.disabilityscoop.com/2014/10/21/feds-schools-bullying/19775/

Chapter 8
Bullying and Victimization of Youth in the Court Systems

Abstract In Chap. 8, we discuss how and why youth who are involved in the juvenile justice system and child welfare system are prone to bullying and peer victimization. Research suggests that youth who are detained in juvenile correctional facilities are seriously at risk of bullying and peer victimization as these youth have opportunities to affiliate with peers who engage in such behavior. Although research on bullying involvement of adolescents in the child welfare system is rare, youth who are placed in out-of-home care (e.g., foster care, kinship care, group home, or residential treatment facility) are also prone to bullying and victimization, as they are typically removed from their home due to allegations of maltreatment; as a result, these youths are likely to have difficulty in socialization and forming bonds with "conventional" peers and are likely to be victimized or socially excluded.

Keywords Delinquency · Juvenile justice · Child welfare system

Introduction

In this chapter, we explore the experiences in bullying and peer victimization of children and adolescents who are involved in the court system, namely, juvenile justice and child welfare systems. As numerous research has shown, youth who are delinquent are at significant risk of being involved in the juvenile justice system and are significantly more at risk of engaging in bullying compared to their peers who are not involved in the juvenile justice system. Similarly, despite the few available research on bullying involvement of children and adolescents in the child welfare system, some studies have been conducted outside the United States, such as Croatia. Studies in Croatia, for instance, have documented that youth in residential care are significantly likely to be involved in bullying incidents, both as a victim and as a perpetrator. In this chapter, we first discuss the relevance of juvenile justice and child welfare systems in bullying and peer victimization of adolescents involved in these systems. Next, we discuss the relevance of delinquency and child welfare involvement in adolescents' experiences in bullying through a social-ecological framework.

A. A. Peguero, J. S. Hong, *School Bullying*, Springer Series on Child and Family Studies, https://doi.org/10.1007/978-3-030-64367-6_8

Delinquency and Juvenile Justice System

Juvenile delinquency, conceptualized as minors engaging in behaviors or acts that are considered illegal [1], has prompted policymakers to come up with specific and detailed procedures for addressing criminal activities that are committed by minors. In the 1990s, almost every state in the United States had enacted punitive measures to address delinquency, and most states had limited juvenile court jurisdictions over to the adult criminal justice systems for serious and heinous offenses, such as murder and rape [2]. Juvenile delinquency has also been implicated in research on risk factors for bullying. While a great deal of research literature showed that bullying perpetration and bullying victimization are significant risk factors that are positively associated with delinquent behaviors [3–6], some studies also found that adolescents who participate in delinquent behaviors are also likely to be at an increased risk of participating in bullying and antisocial behaviors [7, 8].

Several theories shed light on the association between juvenile delinquency and bullying behavior. Social learning theorists, for example, argue that delinquent adolescents are likely to affiliate with peers who engage in similar behaviors, and are likely to repeat such behavior as a result. According to the social learning theory, adolescents who affiliate with delinquent and antisocial peer groups are likely to observe and model such behaviors, which can increase aggressive and bullying behaviors. The attachment theorist also may posit that youth who did not have a secure attachment with their primary caregivers are at an increased risk of turning to delinquent peers; as a result, these youth are likely to become delinquent and act aggressively towards their peers. The general strain theorists on the other hand postulate that strainful relationships (e.g., bullying victimization) can contribute to stress, which can pressure adolescents into criminal and delinquent acts [9]. According to Cullen, Unnever, Hartman, Turner, and Agnew [10], victims of bullying also showed a significant risk of delinquent behaviors, and the effect of victimization on delinquency was particularly strong among adolescents who had weaker bonds with social institutions (e.g., school) and with high levels of aggressive attitudes.

Child Welfare System

According to Child Trends [11], there was a significant increase in the number of children in out-of-home care, from 567,000 in 1999 to 443,000 in 2017. Also, according to the U.S. Department of Health and Human Services [12], in 2016, 437,465 children and adolescents who were placed in foster care. A child enters foster care or other out-of-home care arrangements when a child welfare worker (e.g., child protective services worker) determines that it is unsafe for the child to remain at his or her home due to a risk of maltreatment. Out-of-home care placement and services (foster home, kinship, or relatives' homes, group or residential care or institutions) are provided to children who are removed from their home because of safety concerns. Interestingly, research findings showed that among children in out-of-home care, the risk of victimization perpetrated by peers was higher than the risk of victimization by adults [13, 14]. Empirical studies have explored the experiences in bullying and victimization of adolescents involved in the child welfare system are limited. Despite the paucity of empirical evidence, peer victimization is frequent and severe among children who are placed in out-of-home care, which is highly likely to be based on racial or ethnic differences, cultural differences, religious differences, actual or perceived sexual orientation, disability status, low self-esteem, and unique family structure [15]. For instance, according to the American Bar Association [16], almost all children in group homes who are lesbian, gay, bisexual, and transgender reported experiencing verbal harassment by their peers, and 70% of these children were victims of violence perpetrated by their peers. Other studies also found that as many as 30% of out-of-home care children had reported being victimized by their peers [e.g., 17]. The Child Welfare League of America [18] reported from an informal survey conducted by FosterClub of former foster youth that over half of the respondents reported being victimized by their peers because they were in the foster care system. Numerous empirical studies in several different countries had documented the severity of bullying among children involved in the child welfare system. In one research, which investigated bullying perpetration and victimization rates among adolescent girls in the child welfare system, girls in the child welfare system were significantly more likely to bully others or be bullied by their peers relative to those who were not involved in the child welfare system [19]. Findings from another research by Mohapatra and colleagues [20] in Canada also indicated that adolescents whose family were involved in child protection services were more likely to experience and engage in bullying than their peers who were not involved in child protective services. Research by Kim and colleagues [21], which included South Korean elementary school students in the child welfare system, found that 22% of the students in a lower grade and 12% of the students in the higher group reported experiencing peer victimization. The study also found that children involved in bullying reported internalizing and externalizing problems, including somatization, depressive symptoms, attention deficit hyperactive disorder, internet addiction, and suicidal ideation. Although bullying and teasing are prevalent and constitute a serious problem for children involved in the child welfare system, these children have fewer supports available.

Children in out-of-home care children are especially vulnerable to peer victimization because they frequently move to different classrooms or schools, which affords them fewer opportunities to develop friendships supportive peer networks, making them easy targets for peer victimization [15]. Moreover, peer group hierarchies or "pecking orders" are a central context in which peer victimization is experienced by out-of-home care children. Barter's [22] qualitative study, for example, found that children who were placed in a residential care facility bullied new residents in an effort to maintain their power and status. Further, school districts treat out-of-home care students with less concern than students in the general population, as school officials are likely to perceive out-of-home care students as "transplanted problems" [15]. Regrettably, there is a serious dearth of training for teachers and school administrators to effectively recognize the needs of children involved in the child welfare system.

Social-Ecological Framework

In this section, we present the significance of youths' involvement in both the juvenile justice system and child welfare system and how they relate to bullying victimization and perpetration through a social-ecological framework, which consists of societal, community, institutional, group, and individual-level factors.

Societal

Although there appears to be a dearth of empirical evidence, bullying involvement of youth with delinquent behaviors appears to be a by-product of the current measures that convict juvenile offenders as adults. Following the tough-on-crime period, the practice of trying minors as adults for heinous crimes became more frequent [23], and between 1990 and 2010, the number of minors in the adult criminal justice system had soared exponentially. Opponents of the existing juvenile justice system argue that youth who are confined in adult facilities encounter grave danger to their safety, as they are likely to experience higher rates of physical and sexual abuse by adults. Juvenile offenders who are locked up in adult prisons are at significant risk of being bullied by adult inmates who are usually physically stronger, have a long criminal history, and have more experiences with being in a correctional facility [24]. Moreover, youths who are confined in an adult correctional facility have numerous opportunities to observe and model aggressive behavior from adult inmates, which can increase their opportunities to misbehave and display bullying and aggressive behavior. One descriptive study of bullying in prisons reported a high percentage of bullying experienced by inmates [25], and adolescents who are confined in an adult prison setting have a high risk of developing bullying and aggressive behaviors.

With respect to child welfare, historically, the child welfare system has not been held accountable for the developmental, mental health, and school outcomes of children in the system [26], which might be attributed to a lack of comprehensive measures. Moreover, a lack of early comprehensive developmental, mental health, and educational assessments for healthy functioning [26] can result in peer conflicts, bullying, and fighting among children in the child welfare system. Children and adolescents in the child welfare system, such as the foster care system are given limited opportunities to interact with other children in the foster care system, which reflects a major dearth of systematic programs that are inclusive of all children in foster care [26]. Consequently, these children are frequently and continuously marginalized and feel socially isolated because they are unable to relate to their peers in school, which is likely to increase their odds of being victimized or socially excluded by their classmates and peers.

Community

Juvenile delinquency affects not only those involved but also the entire community. For instance, exposure to violence in the community can affect adolescents at risk of delinquent behavior, which can subsequently affect the community-at-large. As research has shown, youth who are exposed to violence in their community on a daily bases are especially likely to participate in delinquent and deviant behaviors [27, 28], such as violent offending [29]. Among youth who are at risk of delinquency, consistent exposure to community violence can result in learned aggressive behaviors [30], as explained by the social learning theory. In a violent social environment, youth who frequently witness or experience community violence might be predisposed to bullying and assaultive behaviors in an effort to garner respect from their peers [31]. Also, exposure to community violence can increase adolescents' risk of victimization by their peers. As argued by routine activities theorists, the movement of activities in the community provides opportunities for victimization. The routine activities theories consist of three components, such as (1) motivated offenders (perpetrators), (2) suitable targets (victims), and (3) absence of capable guardians. Delinquent youth who are engaged in activities (e.g., delinquency) in the community among peers and out of control of parents or other capable adults become easy targets of victimization [29], particularly victimization by their peers.

Research conducted over the years has consistently shown a link between deteriorating neighborhood conditions and children's involvement in the child welfare system, which is largely because of maltreatment [32]. Neighborhood conditions, such as poverty in the neighborhood, for example, can increase children's chance of being maltreatment, which results in being placed in an alternative care setting, such as foster home, group home, or residential care facility. Adolescents with a history of childhood maltreatment in an alternative care setting encounter several challenges, such as difficulty in forming friendships and in relating with their peers, which increases their likelihood of being victimized or socially excluded by their peer groups. Further, these adolescents likely follow pathways from emotional dysregulation to a display of antisocial behavior [33] and other externalizing behaviors [34], which are likely to result in bullying involvement. The relationship between childhood maltreatment and bullying behavior is also consistent with the social learning theory; that is, maltreated adolescents observe and model aggressive behavior of their parents. Also, the attachment theory would posit that maltreated adolescents do not form a secure attachment with their primary caregiver (e.g., biological parents), and consequently, they have difficulty in socialization and relating to others (e.g., peers [35]), possibly leading to peer victimization.

Institutional

Bullying and aggressive behaviors can create a climate of fear in institutions, such as juvenile detention centers, as a youth in detention centers are consistently exposed to other at-risk youth who display such behaviors. Youth in detention centers commonly had previously experienced multiple stressors, such as victimization (e.g., abuse in the home, bullying by peers, exposure to community violence), which can lead to traumatic stressors. "[T]raumatic stressors are events that involve a threat, or the actual occurrence of an untimely death or severe physical injury that could be life threatening, or a violation of bodily integrity (i.e., sexual assault or molestation" [36, p. 694]. In the United States, more than 75% of adolescents had reported going through at least one type of trauma-related stress in their lifetime [37]. For youth in a juvenile detention facility, traumatic stressors can elicit aggressive attitudes and behavior [36]. Disruptions in the attachment with a primary caregiver frequently happen when youth are frequently removed from the biological family, putting them at a heightened risk for more complex trauma and subsequently, reinforcing aggressive behavior [38].

Various institutions, such as schools, mental health institutions, and residential care facilities can increase bullying and peer victimization of adolescents in the child welfare system, such as foster care. School districts, for example, can create an uncomfortable school environment for children who are removed from their biological families, which can reinforce trauma and other behavioral problems [15]. Many foster parents also described how foster care children are not readily accepted by their classmates and peers, which can make them vulnerable to peer victimization. Further, children who are in the child welfare system demonstrate a serious need for, and use of mental health-related services [39], especially for depression PTSD, ADHD, and substance use, which are positively related to childhood abuse and are likely to lead to peer relationship problems, such as bullying and peer victimization [40]. Also, with regards to bullying involvement of adolescents placed in residential care facilities, the residential facility can increase bullying incidents through an invasion of personal space, detachment from support networks, cultures of non-disclosure, and attacks at night [41].

Group

Bullying is not merely a dyadic problem that only involves the perpetrator and the target; rather, it is a group phenomenon, which occurs in a social context in which a variety of factors might encourage, maintain, or inhibit such behavior [42, 43]. As purported by Salmivalli [44], bullying is a "group process" involving a group of adolescents picking on an individual. Also, during adolescence, youth increasingly turn to their peer groups and spend a large amount of time with their peer groups. In juvenile detention facilities, deviant peer group affiliation and gang affiliation are serious concerns [45], and adolescents who are involved in these affiliations are likely to develop antisocial behavior and engage in bullying. In one study, including a sample of youth in a juvenile detention facility, 64% (n = 87) were found to be identified as having "high-risk" gang norms, and 36% were identified as having "low-risk" gang norms [46]. Adolescents confined in a juvenile detention facility may choose to associate with deviant peer groups or a gang because they feel not having a place to belong or perceive their affiliates as a source of protection from bullying and harassment [see 47].

Research to date has yet to investigate a possible association between types of out-of-home placement to gang affiliation, although youth placed in an out-of-home setting, in general, are shown at an increased likelihood of participating in delinquent activities [48–50], which is also likely to increase their risk of gang affiliation and bullying and peer victimization. From a large sample of adolescents in kinship care placements, Ryan and colleagues [48] reported that the relative risk of delinquency was significantly higher in adolescents in a kinship placement and group home placement. Ryan and colleagues' [49] study also reported that the relative risk of delinquency was significantly greater for adolescents placed in a group home compared to those placed in a foster home. Youth in out-of-home care commonly report feeling marginalized, as they have difficulty in establishing a friendship with "conventional" peer groups; According to the multiple marginality perspective, youth in out-of-home care experience numerous social and economic disadvantage, which can diminish their educational and social functioning, pushing them towards peers who are involved in deviant and delinquent behavior and street life and "street socialization" [51].

Individual

Individual-level factors relevant to adolescent bullying and peer victimization have been examined extensively in research [see 52]. Research on bullying has examined, particular ontological correlates, most notably, sex and race/ethnicity (see Chaps. 4 and 5). According to the National Center for Education Statistics of the Bureau of Justice, a higher percentage of females reported peer victimization [53], which was contrary to empirical findings. Research consistently shows that bullying, particularly physical and verbal-types of bullying, is much higher among males [54, 55]. Findings on racial differences in bullying have been inconsistent. As reported by the NCES, White/European Americans (24%) were the highest racial group who reported victimization. Among other racial and ethnic groups, a higher percentage of Black/African Americans reported being victimized than Hispanic/Latino Americans or Asian Americans [53]. However, empirical findings on racial and ethnic differences in bullying are largely inconsistent. To illustrate, Spriggs, Iannotti, Nansel, and Haynie [56] reported that African Americans had a considerably lower rate of peer victimization than White/European Americans and Hispanic/Latinos. On the other hand, Wang and colleagues' [55] study found that African

Americans were most likely to be identified as bullies and least likely to identify as victims, relative to their peers of other racial and ethnic groups. Peguero's [57] study, however, revealed that Hispanic/Latino Americans and Asian Americans are at an elevated risk of peer victimization, while Juvonen, Graham, and Schuster [58] reported that White/European Americans are most likely while Hispanic/Latino Americans are least likely to experience or participate in peer bullying.

Concerning adolescents involved in the juvenile justice system, the research literature has also examined sex and racial/ethnic differences in delinquent behaviors. While some studies reported a higher rate of males who engage in delinquent behavior [e.g., 59], others have reported no significant sex differences in the patterns of delinquency [e.g., 60]. Males have long been considered to be "aggressive sex" and are arrested more often than females. Also, female delinquent behaviors had largely been considered unimportant; however, interest in female delinquency has increased because the rate of female delinquent behavior has risen over the years. Regarding racial and ethnic differences, racial and ethnic minority adolescents, particularly African American youth, are found to be overrepresented in each and every stage of the juvenile justice system—arrest, adjudication, confinement, and transfer to the adult criminal justice system [61, 62]. The issue of disproportionate minority confinement in the U.S. juvenile justice system remains a growing and serious concern among researchers, policymakers, and youth advocates [63].

According to the Annie E. Casey Foundation [64], despite the narrowed gender gap in a foster care placement from 2008 to 2017 [64], a higher percentage of males are placed in foster care. These data are expected given that boys are significantly more likely than girls to be physically abused at home by their primary caregivers and are most frequently placed in out-of-home care as a result. Moreover, as of September 30, 2016, of the 437,465 children placed in foster care, 44% were identified as White, 23% were identified as Black/African American, 21% were identified as Hispanic/Latino American, and 9% were identified as other races or multiracial [65]. Research shows a disproportionate representation of racial and ethnic minority children's involvement in the child welfare system [12], and minority children are significantly more likely to stay in foster care longer than White/European American children [66, 67].

Based on the aforementioned findings, although research evidence remains inconclusive, it appears that bullying and peer victimization might be more frequent among male and racial and ethnic minority adolescents who have been involved in the juvenile justice system as well as the child welfare system.

Complexities

Several complexities need to be mentioned when understanding the experiences of bullying and peer victimization of adolescents in the juvenile justice and child welfare systems. In this chapter, we focused on delinquent behavior in general, although "delinquency" encompasses, various types of acts ranging from serious offenses, such as homicide to less serious offenses, such as shoplifting. Youth in the juvenile justice system for a serious offense may be more likely to exhibit bullying and aggressive behaviors relative to those who are incarcerated for minor offenses, particularly "victim-less" offenses. In terms of child welfare involvement, as previously mentioned, the research literature on bullying and victimization of adolescents in the child welfare system is quite limited. Similar to involvement in the juvenile justice system, out-of-home placement varies; adolescents in the child welfare system who are in out-of-home care are typically placed in foster care, kinship foster care, group home, or residential treatment facility. The dynamics of peer interaction and socialization might differ, depending on where the youth is placed. For instance, an adolescent's relations with their peers in group homes, which provide a "home-like" treatment setting to a small group of youth, are likely to be different from those in a foster care or kinship care setting. It is also possible that because of the greater frequency of peer interactions in a group home or a residential treatment facility, bullying may be more frequent in these settings.

Males are shown to have a greater propensity for bullying, as they are also more likely to be involved in both juvenile justice and child welfare systems, relative to their female counterparts. However, it is important to mention that the intersecting role of sex/gender in court involvement and bullying dynamics is complex. Over the years, research has concluded that the gender gap in bullying and involvement in the juvenile justice and child welfare systems narrowed over the years. Females are as likely as males to bully their peers, and the rate of females involved in the juvenile justice system has surged over the years. Although pas research has reported that boys prone to direct forms of bullying (physical and verbal) and girls tend to engage in indirect forms of bullying (e.g., relational aggression) [68], an increasing amount of studies are reporting little or no gender differences in bullying and victimization [69].

Concerning racial and ethnic differences in bullying, the juvenile justice system, and the child welfare system, scholars have pointed out the racial disproportionality in the current system. For instance, Black/African American adolescents have been reported to participate in bullying more frequently than their peers of other racial and ethnic groups; they also have a higher likelihood of being involved in the juvenile justice and the court systems than their White/European American peers. The overrepresentation of racial minorities in the court system is reflective of the structural factors, such as poverty, exposure to crime and violence in the neighborhood, and racism in the justice system, which might increase their risk of not only bullying perpetration but also victimization by their peers. For racial and ethnic minorities, they may display aggressive behavior in an effort to protect themselves from the dangers and injustice they are confronted with daily. Although many studies have examined racial differences in bullying and victimization (see Chap. 5), scholars must consider how racial and ethnic minorities, particularly those who live in poverty, cope with the daily stressors they are faced with.

Conclusion

In this chapter, we aimed to explore bullying and peer victimization of adolescents in the juvenile justice system and those in the child welfare system. In particular, we attempted to demonstrate that bullying and peer victimization of adolescents in the court systems also need to be understood within the societal, institutional, community, group, and individual contexts in the United States. Considering that empirical literature of bullying experiences of court-involved youth, particularly those in the child welfare system is seriously limited, additional research needs to be conducted to investigate risk factors, as well as protective factors that are associated with bullying and victimization. More importantly, intervention and treatment for youth in the court system need to be relevant to their sex and racial/ethnic identity, as bullying and victimization might be increased when we consider their minoritized status.

References

1. Siegel, L. J., & Welsh, B. C. (2011). *Juvenile delinquency: The core* (4th ed.). Belmont, CA: Wadsworth/Cengage Learning.
2. Blackburn, S. (2019). Juvenile justice in Pennsylvania: Mission-driven; performance-based; outcome-focused. *Juvenile and Family Court Journal, 70*(1), 73–87.
3. Bender, D., & Lösel, F. (2011). Bullying at school as a predictor of delinquency, violence and other anti-social behaviour in adulthood. *Criminal Behaviour and Mental Health, 21*(2), 99–106.
4. Farrington, D. P., Loeber, R., Stallings, R., & Ttofi, M. M. (2011). Bullying perpetration and victimization as predictors of delinquency and depression in the Pittsburgh Youth Study. *Journal of Aggression, Conflict and Peace Research, 3*, 74.
5. Higgins, G. E., Khey, D. N., Dawson-Edwards, B. C., & Marcum, C. D. (2012). Examining the link between being a victim of bullying and delinquency trajectories among an African American sample. *International Criminal Justice Review, 22*(2), 110–122.
6. McCuddy, T., & Esbensen, F.-A. (2017). After the bell and into the night: The link between delinquency and traditional, cyber-, and dual-bullying victimization. *Journal of Research in Crime and Delinquency, 54*(3), 409–441.
7. Ireland, J. L., & Archer, J. (2004). Association between measures of aggression and bullying among juvenile and young offenders. *Aggressive Behavior, 30*(1), 29–42.
8. Wiklund, G., Ruchkin, V. V., Koposov, R. A., & af Klinteberg, B. (2014). Pro-bullying attitudes among incarcerated juvenile delinquents: Antisocial behavior, psychopathic tendencies and violent crime. *International Journal of Law and Psychiatry, 37*(3), 281–288.
9. Hay, C., & Meldrum, R. (2010). Bullying victimization and adolescent self-harm: Testing hypotheses from general strain theory. *Journal of Youth and Adolescence, 39*(5), 446–459.
10. Cullen, F. T., Unnever, J. D., Hartman, J. L., Turner, M. G., & Agnew, R. (2008). Gender, bullying victimization, and juvenile delinquency: A test of general strain theory. *Victims and Offenders, 3*(4), 346–364.
11. Child Trends. (2018). *Foster Care*. Child Trends. Retrieved August 18, 2020, from https://www.childtrends.org/indicators/foster-care.
12. U.S. Department of Health and Human Services. (2017). The AFCARS Report. Retrieved from https://www.acf.hhs.gov/sites/default/files/cb/afcarsreport24.pdf

13. Farmer, E., & Pollock, S. (1998). *Sexually abused and abusing children in substitute care*. Chichester: John Wiley.
14. Sinclair, I., & Gibbs, I. (1998). *Children's homes: A study in diversity*. Chichester: John Wiley.
15. Vacca, J. S., & Kramer-Vida, L. (2012). Preventing the bullying of foster children in our schools. *Children and Youth Services Review, 34*(9), 1805–1809.
16. American Bar Association (n.d.). Resolution 107A unanimously approved by the ABA House of Delegates. Retrieved from http://www.civilrights.org/assets/pdfs/aba-
17. Rao, V., & Simkiss, D. (2007). Bullying in schools: A survey of the experience of looked after children. *Adoption & Fostering, 31*(3), 49–57.
18. Child Welfare League of America. (n.d.). Is bullying a form of abuse? CWLA's Children's Voice magazine examines issues including impact on foster children. Retrieved from http://www.cwla.org/newsevents/news2011039bully.htm
19. Sterzing, P. R., Auslander, W. F., Ratliff, G. A., Gerke, D. R., Edmond, T., & Jonson-Reid, M. (2020). Exploring bullying perpetration and victimization among adolescent girls in the child welfare system: Bully-only, victim-only, bully-victim, and noninvolved roles. *Journal of Interpersonal Violence, 35*(5–6), 1311–1333.
20. Mohapatra, S., Irving, H., Paglia-Boak, A., Wekerle, C., Adlaf, E., & Rehm, J. (2010). History of family involvement with child protective services as a risk factor for bullying in Ontario schools. *Child and Adolescent Mental Health, 15*(3), 157–163.
21. Kim, J. W., Lee, K., Lee, Y. S., Han, D. H., Min, K. J., Song, S. H., Kim, J. O., et al. (2015). Factors associated with group bullying and psychopathology in elementary school students using child-welfare facilities. *Neuropsychiatric Disease and Treatment, 11*, 991.
22. Barter, C. (2003). Young people in residential care talk about peer violence. *Scottish Journal of Residential Child Care, 2*, 39–50.
23. Shook, J. J., & Sarri, R. C. (2008). Trends in the committee of juveniles to adult prisons: Toward an increased willingness to treat juveniles as adults. *The Wayne Law Review, 54*, 1725.
24. Lambie, I., & Randell, I. (2013). The impact of incarceration on juvenile offenders. *Clinical Psychology Review, 33*(3), 448–459.
25. Ireland, J., & Archer, J. (1996). Descriptive analysis of bullying in male and female adult prisoners. *Journal of Community & Applied Social Psychology, 6*(1), 35–47.
26. Bruskas, D. (2008). Children in foster care: A vulnerable population at risk. *Journal of Child and Adolescent Psychiatric Nursing, 21*(2), 70–77.
27. Herrenkohl, T. I., Hawkins, J. D., Chung, I., Hill, K. G., & Battin-Pearson, S. (2001). School and community risk factors and interventions. In R. Loeber & D. P. Farrington (Eds.), *Child delinquents: Development, intervention, and service needs* (pp. 211–246). Thousand Oaks, CA: Sage.
28. Patchin, J. W., Huebner, B. M., McCluskey, J. D., Varano, S. P., & Bynum, T. S. (2006). Exposure to community violence and childhood delinquency. *Crime & Delinquency, 52*(2), 307–332.
29. Nofziger, S., & Kurtz, D. (2005). Violent lives: A lifestyle model linking exposure to violence to juvenile violent offending. *Journal of Research in Crime and Delinquency, 42*(1), 3–26.
30. Agnew, R. (2002). Experienced, vicarious, and anticipated strain: An exploratory study on physical victimization and delinquency. *Justice Quarterly, 19*(4), 603–632.
31. Anderson, E. (1999). *Code of the street: Decency, violence, and the moral life of the inner city*. New York: Norton.
32. Rolock, N., Jantz, I., & Abner, K. (2015). Community perceptions and foster care placement: A multi-level analysis. *Children and Youth Services Review, 48*, 186–191.
33. Jaffee, S. R., Caspi, A., Moffitt, T. E., & Taylor, A. (2004). Physical maltreatment victim to antisocial child: Evidence of an environmentally mediated process. *Journal of Abnormal Psychology, 113*(1), 44.
34. Heleniak, C., Jenness, J. L., Vander Stoep, A., McCauley, E., & McLaughlin, K. A. (2016). Childhood maltreatment exposure and disruptions in emotion regulation: A transdiagnostic pathway to adolescent internalizing and externalizing psychopathology. *Cognitive Therapy and Research, 40*(3), 394–415.

35. Howe, T. R., & Parke, R. D. (2001). Friendship quality and sociometric status: Between-group differences and links to loneliness in severely abused and nonabused children. *Child Abuse & Neglect, 25*(5), 585–606.
36. Ford, J. D., Chapman, J., Connor, D. F., & Cruise, K. R. (2012). Complex trauma and aggression in secure juvenile justice settings. *Criminal Justice and Behavior, 39*(6), 694–724.
37. Seedat, S., Nyamai, C., Njenga, F., Vythilingum, B., & Stein, D. J. (2004). Trauma exposure and post-traumatic stress symptoms in urban African schools: Survey in Cape Town and Nairobi. *The British Journal of Psychiatry, 184*(2), 169–175.
38. Ford, J. D., Connor, D. F., & Hawke, J. (2009). Complex trauma among psychiatrically impaired children: A cross-sectional, chart-review study. *The Journal of Clinical Psychiatry, 70*, 1155.
39. Shin, S. H. (2005). Need for and actual use of mental health service by adolescents in the child welfare system. *Children and Youth Services Review, 27*(10), 1071–1083.
40. Sterzing, P. R., Auslander, W. F., & Goldbach, J. T. (2014). An exploratory study of bullying involvement for sexual minority youth: Bully-only, victim-only, and bully-victim roles. *Journal of the Society for Social Work and Research, 5*(3), 321–337.
41. Monks, C. P., Smith, P. K., Naylor, P., Barter, C., Ireland, J. L., & Coyne, I. (2009). Bullying in different contexts: Commonalities, differences and the role of theory. *Aggression and Violent Behavior, 14*(2), 146–156.
42. Olweus, D. (2001). Peer harassment: A critical analysis and some important questions. In J. Juvonen & S. Graham (Eds.), *Peer harassment in school: The plight of the vulnerable and victimized* (pp. 3–20). New York, NY: Guilford Press.
43. Rodkin, P. C., & Hodges, E. V. (2003). Bullies and victims in the peer ecology: Four questions for psychologists and school professionals. *School Psychology Review, 32*(3), 384–400.
44. Salmivalli, C. (2010). Bullying and the peer group: A review. *Aggression and Violent Behavior, 15*(2), 112–120.
45. Egley, A., Jr., & Arjunan, M. (2002). *Highlights of the 2000 National Youth Gang Survey (Fact Sheet# 04)*. Washington, DC: Office of Juvenile Justice and Delinquency Prevention.
46. King, K. M., Voisin, D. R., & DiClemente, R. J. (2013). Gang norms and risky sex among adolescents with a history of detention. *Journal of Social Service Research, 39*(4), 545–551.
47. Hess, K. M., Orthmann, C. H., & Wright, J. P. (2013). *Juvenile justice*. Belmont, CA: Cengage Learning.
48. Ryan, J. P., Hong, J. S., Herz, D., & Hernandez, P. M. (2010). Kinship foster care and the risk of juvenile delinquency. *Children and Youth Services Review, 32*(12), 1823–1830.
49. Ryan, J. P., Marshall, J. M., Herz, D., & Hernandez, P. M. (2008). Juvenile delinquency in child welfare: Investigating group home effects. *Children and Youth Services Review, 30*(9), 1088–1099.
50. Ryan, J. P., Testa, M. F., & Zhai, F. (2008). African American males in foster care and the risk of delinquency: The value of social bonds and permanence. *Child Welfare, 87*(1), 115.
51. Vigil, J. D. (2010). *Barrio gangs: Street life and identity in Southern California*. Austin, TX: University of Texas Press.
52. Hong, J. S., & Espelage, D. L. (2012). A review of research on bullying and peer victimization in school: An ecological system analysis. *Aggression and Violent Behavior, 17*(4), 311–322.
53. Robers, S., Zhang, A., & Morgan, R. E. (2015). Indicators of School Crime and Safety: 2014. NCES 2015-072/NCJ 248036. *National Center for Education Statistics*.
54. Griffiths, L. J., Wolke, D., Page, A. S., & Horwood, J. (2006). Obesity and bullying: Different effects for boys and girls. *Archives of Disease in Childhood, 91*(2), 121–125.
55. Wang, J., Iannotti, R. J., & Nansel, T. R. (2009). School bullying among adolescents in the United States: Physical, verbal, relational, and cyber. *Journal of Adolescent Health, 45*(4), 368–375.
56. Spriggs, A. L., Iannotti, R. J., Nansel, T. R., & Haynie, D. L. (2007). Adolescent bullying involvement and perceived family, peer and school relations: Commonalities and differences across race/ethnicity. *Journal of Adolescent Health, 41*(3), 283–293.

57. Peguero, A. A. (2009). Victimizing the children of immigrants: Latino and Asian American student victimization. *Youth & Society, 41*(2), 186–208.
58. Juvonen, J., Graham, S., & Schuster, M. A. (2003). Bullying among young adolescents: The strong, the weak, and the troubled. *Pediatrics, 112*(6), 1231–1237.
59. Herrera, V. M., & McCloskey, L. A. (2001). Gender differences in the risk for delinquency among youth exposed to family violence☆,☆☆. *Child Abuse & Neglect, 25*(8), 1037–1051.
60. Liu, X., & Kaplan, H. B. (1999). Explaining the gender difference in adolescent delinquent behavior: A longitudinal test of mediating mechanisms. *Criminology, 37*(1), 195–216.
61. Bishop, D. M. (2005). The role of race and ethnicity in juvenile justice processing. In D. F. Hawkins & K. Kempf-Leonard (Eds.), *Our children, their children: Confronting racial and ethnic differences in American juvenile justice* (pp. 23–82). Chicago, IL: University of Chicago Press.
62. Sickmund, M. (2009). Delinquency cases in juvenile court, 2005. *Drugs, 17*, 20.
63. Davis, J., & Sorensen, J. R. (2013). Disproportionate minority confinement of juveniles: A national examination of Black–White disparity in placements, 1997–2006. *Crime & Delinquency, 59*(1), 115–139.
64. Annie E. Casey Foundation (2020). Kids count data center. Retrieved August 19, 2020, from https://datacenter.kidscount.org/data/tables/6245-children-in-foster-care-by-gender
65. Children's Bureau (n.d.). Foster care statistics 2017. Retrieved from https://www.childwelfare.gov/pubPDFs/foster.pdf
66. Hill, R. B. (2005). The role of race in parental reunification. In D. M. Derezotes, J. Poetner, & M. F. Testa (Eds.), *Race matters in child welfare: The overrepresentation of African American children in the system* (pp. 215–230). Washington, DC: CWLA Press.
67. Hill, R. B. (2006). Synthesis of Research on Disproportionality in Child Welfare: An Update. Washington DC: Casey-CSSP Alliance for Racial Equity in the Child Welfare System, 2006. Retrieved from http://www.caseyfamilyservices.org/pdfs/0226_CC_BobHillPaper_FINAL.pdf
68. Putallaz, M., Grimes, C. L., Foster, K. J., Kupersmidt, J. B., Coie, J. D., & Dearing, K. (2007). Overt and relational aggression and victimization: Multiple perspectives within the school setting. *Journal of School Psychology, 45*(5), 523–547.
69. Barboza, G. E., Schiamberg, L. B., Oehmke, J., Korzeniewski, S. J., Post, L. A., & Heraux, C. G. (2009). Individual characteristics and the multiple contexts of adolescent bullying: An ecological perspective. *Journal of Youth and Adolescence, 38*(1), 101–121.

Chapter 9
Conclusion: Implications and Addressing School Bullying and Inequality

Abstract In the concluding Chap. 9, we discuss why ameliorating violence and victimization should be a priority. Of course, addressing bullying victimization that occurs within schools for all youth is paramount toward sustaining a system that is supposed to facilitate educational progress and sustainability. There is a persistent history of disparities linked to socioeconomic and social status, family cohesion and interactions, sexual orientation, gender identity, and gender expression, race, ethnicity, immigration, and religion, and disabilities and special health needs in the U.S. school system. The social problem of bullying within U.S. schools is both complex and diverse. It is clear that the sources and factors associated with the vulnerability and marginalization of youth to being victimized at school presented in this book also intersect. Although homes, schools, and neighborhoods may never be completely bully-free environments, there are several ways to assist students in breaking the bullying and peer victimization cycles. The information presented in this book is also one calling for advocacy, which will suggest that if policymakers, school administrators, and community stakeholders are seeking to address and ameliorate bullying within schools, it is vital to consider the significance of various forms of social inequality.

Keywords Bullying prevention · Theoretical implications · Policy implications

Introduction

In this concluding chapter, we discuss the implications of and how to address social inequality (i.e., socioeconomic and social status, family cohesion and interactions, sex, sexual orientation, gender identity, and gender expression, race, ethnicity, immigration, and religion, disabilities and special health needs, and court involvement) with school bullying. As discussed throughout this book, most school bullying research has focused on the differential patterns of victimization. In this book, however, we have presented the importance of considering inequality when understanding, researching, and addressing school bullying. In this chapter, we will first discuss the implications of the role inequality should have as educational faculty,

A. A. Peguero, J. S. Hong, *School Bullying*, Springer Series on Child and Family Studies, https://doi.org/10.1007/978-3-030-64367-6_9

staff, administrators, and policymakers seek to address and ameliorate bullying for marginalized and vulnerable youth in U.S. schools. We then discuss the implications of inequality for commonly practiced school safety and anti-bullying policies such as zero-tolerance and social control, Schoolwide Positive Behavioral Interventions and Supports programs (SWBIS), communal schools, Olweus bullying prevention, and restorative justice programs. We then highlight the importance of considering the symbiotic relationship between educational success, progress, and well-being with the safety of marginalized and vulnerable youth in U.S. schools. We then conclude with some final takeaways from this book toward understanding, researching, and addressing school bullying and inequality.

Implications for Educational Faculty, Staff, Administrators, and Policymakers

Throughout this book, we have highlighted how the U.S. socio-political landscape contextualizes the social inequality of bullying and the lives of marginalized and vulnerable youth. Researchers have suggested that because differential privilege is perpetuated by the process of schooling, teachers, and administrators committed to educational equality and providing healthy and safe learning environments must take responsibility. This means that school personnel should consider the role of social inequality in association with their behaviors, actions, stereotypical images and myths, and policy enforcement, and to work to change attitudes and practices. School faculty, staff, administrators, and policymakers should prioritize the pursuit of educational equity for disadvantaged and vulnerable students to break the cycle of marginalization. A goal of schools should be to consider implementing practices and policies based on inclusion, empathy, understanding, and protection with their learning as well as socialization.

As presented throughout this book, vulnerable and marginalized students often learn from their teachers and peers that they are "outsiders" and sometimes not welcomed. Vulnerable and marginalized youth have school relationships that are shaped by broader social, cultural, and political discourses and practices on various forms of social inequality. For example, LGBTQ students and their parents were taunted by school staff, teachers, and students who called them homophobic slurs [1–5]. It is also evident that some teachers and administrators punish, discipline, or publicly humiliate LGBTQ students [1, 5, 6]. It is in this type of a school climate, researchers indicate homophobia as an increasing and serious problem for LGBTQ youth in U.S. schools which has detrimental effects on learning and safety [1–5]. In general, teachers and administrators who are concerned with addressing the harassment directed at vulnerable and marginalized students should not only respond to such forms of violence and harassment, they must also be proactive by establishing and sustaining a school climate of inclusion and tolerance.

In multicultural societies, schools play a powerful role in promoting broader, societal discourses that define the necessary qualities and limits of citizenship and social belonging. This suggests that faculty, staff, administrators, and educational policymakers aimed at reducing violence against vulnerable and marginalized youth, as well as ensuring their safety, should recognize the transactions between the macro-political context and micro lived experiences of vulnerable and marginalized youth to create new dispositions and identities, and more inclusive notions of belonging [1, 7, 8]. Without an examination of the relationship between emotions, shifting demographics, and negative embodied practices directed at vulnerable and marginalized students, possibilities for faculty, staff, administrators, and educational policymakers who create healthy climates, equitable schools, and safe classrooms will be lost. Moreover, faculty, staff, administrators, and educational policy makers who continue to separate emotion from pedagogical practices and multicultural competencies are inadequate to address change within an increasingly diverse world. If educators and policymakers wish to prepare faculty, staff, and administrators to challenge and change existing societal inequities for vulnerable and marginalized students, the preparation of school personnel must include opportunities for individual and collective self-reflection and the examination of the blurring of emotions and harassment.

Instead of treating harassment against vulnerable and marginalized youth as a one-off incident that can adequately be addressed through disciplinary sanctions, faculty, staff, administrators, and educational policymakers should prepare students to identify how the broader socio-political context around social inequality can be embodied in the day-to-day interactions of school life, and to explore possibilities that are opened up for interrupting practices that exclude others. Some have proposed that a curriculum of discomfort engages students to analyze the emotional dimensions that frame and shape habits and routines complicit with the marginalization and vulnerabilities endured by disadvantaged students [6, 9, 10]. Preventing violence and harassment against, as well as ensuring the safety of, vulnerable and marginalized students while in school requires educating faculty and administrators to interrogate the feelings that maintain particular forms of relationality between "us" and "them." Educational strategies must be augmented by a consideration of teaching, administrating, counseling, and working with students and families should be "informed by emotion that resists unjust systems and practices as well as emotion that helps create a more fair and just world in our classrooms and everyday lives" [10, p. 174].

Moreover, for harmful actions that maintain boundaries between us and them, educational policymakers should help prospective teachers and administrators recognize the ways that xenophobia, homophobia, sexism, racism, classism, and the like structure their own experiences as well as vulnerable and marginalized youth's experiences at school. Some propose that learning about citizenship occurs in a complex interplay of interests and power would benefit all students [1, 7, 11, 12]. The formation of citizenship identities is socially embedded within learning processes that could facilitate potential teacher and administrator candidates to socialize and educate all students to dismiss or be critical of discourses of exclusion and enhance inclusive interactions and criteria for belonging. For example, on March 23, 2016, an Act to Provide for Single-Sex Multiple Occupancy Bathroom and Changing Facilities in Schools and Public Agencies and to Create Statewide Consistency in Regulation of Employment and Public Accommodations, or what is commonly known as HB2 became law in North Carolina. Prospective teachers and administrators should consider the implications for LGBTQ youth. When such acts are enacted alongside instances of backlash against LGBTQ youth, teachers and administrators could encourage students to question the larger environment, examine the constant dynamic between discourses and practices of exclusion, and produce alternative realities. Thus, in general, educational policymakers who seek to address the violence and harassment against vulnerable and marginalized students in schools should develop a curriculum that trains teachers' and administrators' understanding of larger patterns of exclusion, xenophobia, homophobia, sexism, racism, classism, and the like by fostering democracy and inclusion.

Implications for Zero-Tolerance and Social Control

Foucault [13] is often referred to as conceptualizing this sociological shift toward a "disciplinary society" where he is cited as stating, "factories, schools, barracks, hospitals, which all resemble prisons?" [p. 228]. Moreover, Simon [14] argues that "the technologies, discourses, and metaphors of crime and criminal justice have become more visible features of all kinds of institutions" [p. 4]. These social institutions, including schools, have incorporated policies, mechanisms, techniques, and an overall culture of social control [15–19]. Thus, the influence of governing through crime and violence in nationwide policies, such as a requirement of zero-tolerance policies, as well as financial incentives to schools for police and other security measures, such as those provided in the "Secure Our Schools" Act of 2000 has become a pervasive response to address the public concern and fear of youth violence within schools. As noted, Simon [14] illustrates how governing through violence has influenced rules and practices in schools across social strata; he states that "the very real violence of a few schools concentrated in zones of hardened poverty and social disadvantage has provided a 'truth' of school crime that circulates across whole school systems" [p. 210]. However, there are raising concerns about the expanding use of zero-tolerance and social control within schools because of unintended consequences for youth who attend highly controlled and securitized schools. Research also denotes that surveillance and security, such as police, cameras, and metal detectors create a "prison-like" institutional atmosphere or environment, especially for schools located in disadvantaged or urban areas [15–20].

Although highly securitized schools and zero-tolerance are school safety policies intended to protect students and ensure a safe learning environment, many argue that these social control policies have disproportionately punished vulnerable and marginalized students [15–21]. Disproportionate punishment (e.g., referral, suspension, expulsion) could steer students toward social exclusion, educational failure, and life-long economic hardship [15–21]. Addressing this educational and justice inequality of disproportionate punishment for vulnerable and marginalized students is essential. Of course, we do not discount the argued importance of disciplining adolescents who engage in deviant, delinquent, or violent behavior. However, Muschert and Peguero [22] also argue, "the difficulty in understanding the catalysts for school antiviolence policy development is that the line between caring and undue control is unclear" [p. 123].

There are four recommendations associated with social inequality that should be considered by schools that incorporate zero-tolerance and stringent social control policies. First, administrators should recognize the possibility of criminalization in their efforts to secure school safety. It is not unreasonable to believe that the vulnerable and marginalized students are learning lessons of social inequality. Kupchik [23] stressed that vulnerable and marginalized youth in U.S. schools may be learning the "wrong" lesson when it comes to school discipline practices by suggesting that "this lesson encourages passivity and uncritical acceptance of authority, which bodes poorly for the future of democratic participation" [p. 7]. Thus, faculty, staff, administrators, staff, and security personnel should consider that disadvantaged students are vulnerable to the impact of expulsion and exclusion as they administer sanctions. Second, schools should function and look like educational institutions rather than quasi-prisons. Students recognize larger structural inequalities evident in society, and securitizing schools with metal bars, metal detectors, cameras, and school resource officers creates a disjunction and can alienate students. Worse than alienation, school securitization can lead some students to internalize their role in society as future criminals when they know that schools (like society) cannot trust them to be responsible citizens. Also, when teachers are not focusing on personal safety, teachers can focus on educating students. This is particularly relevant when vulnerable and marginalized students are in heightened fear of their safety while students, faculty, staff, and security personnel use xenophobic, homophobic, sexist, racist, classist, and other forms of biased treatment as a form of control. Third, since security measures can have positive impacts on safety, keeping cameras and surveillance techniques is understandable as a means of monitoring; however, it is encouraged that security guards and school resource officers be trained to understand the complexities and vulnerabilities of disadvantaged youth. As recommended by many, school resource officers should be entering school with specialized training that does not reflect one of crime or social control but rather one of community engagement, conflict resolution, mentoring, and education [22, 24, 25]. Fourth, as noted in this book, vulnerable and marginalized youth and their parents often face socioeconomic, social, cultural, and legal barriers when interacting with school administrators. This can be problematic for school sanctions because contacting and discussing school expulsion and suspension typically requires contacting students' parents; however, faculty, staff, administrators, staff, and security personnel should be thoughtful of socioeconomic, social, cultural, and legal barriers that the parents of vulnerable and marginalized students face when interacting and communicating with school personnel.

Implications for Schoolwide Positive Behavioral Interventions and Supports Programs

Schoolwide Positive Behavior Interventions and Supports (SWPBIS) is a comprehensive and proactive approach to behavior management in schools [26–30]. SWPBIS is being widely disseminated by the U.S. Department of Education and several state departments of education as well as an estimate of more than 9000 schools across the U.S. that implemented this safety policy. SWPBIS is based on the assumption that actively teaching and acknowledging teacher, school, and behavioral expectations can improve the extent to which students expect appropriate behavior from themselves and each other [26–31]. SWPBIS is a universal prevention strategy that aims to alter the school environment by creating improved systems that promote positive change in staff behaviors, which subsequently alter student behaviors. SWPBIS draws on behavioral, social learning, and organizational behavioral principles, which were traditionally used with individual students but have been generalized and applied to an entire student body consistently across all school settings [26–30]. When consistent, positive expectations are established by all adults in a school, the evidence exists that the proportion of students with serious behavior problems will be reduced and the school's overall social climate will improve.

The procedures that define SWPBIS are organized around three main themes: prevention, multi-tiered support, and data-based decision making [26–30]. Investing in the prevention of problem behavior involves: (1) defining and teaching a set of positively stated behavioral expectations to students, teachers and parents (e.g., be safe, respectful, responsible); (2) acknowledging and rewarding those behaviors (e.g., compliance to school rules, safe and respectful peer to peer interactions and academic effort/engagement); (3) systematically supervising students in classrooms and common areas; and (4) establishing and implementing a consistent continuum of corrective consequences for problem behavior. Schools are encouraged to reduce the use of out of class referrals and out of school suspensions as a response to problem behavior [26–30]. The goal is to establish a positive social climate, in which behavioral expectations for students are directly taught, consistently acknowledged, and actively monitored.

There are three recommendations associated with social inequality that should be considered by schools that incorporate SWPBIS practices. First, research suggests that different SWPBIS effects might be observed in schools that are resistant to adopting the model [26–28]. As noted, vulnerable and marginalized students typically attend poorer schools with a higher teacher and administrator turnover; therefore, disadvantaged schools face a serious challenge of having the resources to successfully implement SWPBIS. Second, on a related note, SWPBIS training and sustainability for faculty, staff, and security personnel are vital for program success. Third, implementing school safety practices and rules that are believed to be fair and just by their students are fundamental; however, there is evidence that vulnerable and marginalized students believe that their schools are already unfair and unjust [7, 18, 19, 32–34]. Thus, schools that incorporate SWPBIS should be mindful of the educational inequities vulnerable and marginalized students endure and experience daily.

Implications for Communal Schools

Gottfredson, Payne, and colleagues [35–40] suggest that creating strong communal school organization is an effective, efficient approach toward providing a safe and healthy school climate for students. Defined as the organization of a school as a community, key characteristics include supportive relationships among teachers, administrators, and students all of whom share a common set of goals and norms, collaboration, and involvement [37–40]. Strong communal school organization is found to reduce disorder, violence, and bullying as well as increase academic interest, motivation, and achievement [35–40]. "Healthy" relationships between school administrators, teachers, and students positively influence the climate and effectiveness of that school [35–40]. Schools that implement programs that promote social issues awareness can yield positive results, such as increased school attachment, bonding, attendance, and engagement among all members of the school community [35–40]. School administrators, faculty, and staff who focus on establishing a learning climate that strives for academic excellence often positively influence the school's cultural attitude toward learning. The pursuit of academic excellence is argued to be "contagious" among students, teachers, and administrators in schools that promote such scholastic virtue [35, 36, 38]. The relationships between the school administrators, teachers, staff and students, directly and indirectly, promote learning and safety. Policies and programs that focus on promoting the importance of educational achievement, attainment, and success improve the overall school climate as well as making it safer.

Although there is evidence that communal schools can be effective toward ameliorating violence as well as improving safety, school administrators face several barriers toward establishing communal schools in disadvantaged and urban areas. Even though strong student–teacher relationships, extracurricular activities, and effective collaborations between administrators and faculty can be identified as key elements for communal schools, the resources available to create and sustain a communal school are not always available. High administrator and teacher turnover, limited extracurricular activities, large classrooms, disorder, and low student expectations are historically and persistently evident within disadvantaged and urban schools [41–45]. Although in an ideal sense, communal schools can help establish healthy, safe, and effective learning environments, structural barriers and inequalities restrict stakeholders from building communal schools, particularly in disadvantaged communities.

There are three recommendations associated with social inequality that should be considered by communal schools. First, communal school initiatives should focus on cultural awareness and sensitivity among students. This may be a fruitful avenue for improving school-based safety and fostering the social integration of vulnerable and marginalized students. More specifically, programs that promote open communication among peers and parents of socially and culturally diverse backgrounds, as well as extracurricular activities designed to combat intolerance, are effective at building culturally competent schools [5, 26, 46]. Second, communal school initiatives designed to promote prosocial behavior and student safety must give careful consideration to the changing demographic profile of today's elementary and secondary school populations and the unique challenges faced by vulnerable and marginalized youth. For example, immigrants with limited English proficiency are more likely to report victimization as well as feelings of being unsafe while in school [47–51]. Research suggests that programs aimed at rapid English language acquisition, such as those outlined in *Title III* of the *No Child Left Behind Act*, may improve peer relationships as well as facilitate reporting of violence and victimization. Third, vulnerable and marginalized students' participation in extracurricular activities are often encouraged by school faculty, counselors, and administrators to ameliorate persistent educational inequalities and provide educational opportunities for success [5, 46, 52]. However, as noted in this book, it appears that providing those valuable opportunities, such as academic and athletic extracurricular activities, may be a risk factor for violence and victimization that could negate any educational benefits gained from participation in these activities for vulnerable and marginalized youth. It is important to emphasize that we are not recommending that extracurricular activity involvement should be discouraged. On the contrary, involvement in extracurricular activities has been consistently found to have many educational benefits. What we are suggesting is that administrators and educational policymakers should consider the situational context of students who are involved in these beneficial activities, such as in bands, orchestras, academic clubs, plays, student government, and alike, while considering school policies that attempt to ameliorate students' exposure to school violence and victimization. If a communal school approach is to promote and advocate participation in academic and athletic extracurricular activities as a way to promote or facilitate educational success, addressing the overarching reality of the prevalence of discrimination and educational inequality within the school system must be addressed. Although these initiatives provide a solid footing from which to build more communal schools, there remains a critical dearth of research on how American schools are being reshaped by social and cultural diversity.

Implications for Olweus Bullying Prevention Programs

The Olweus Bullying Prevention Program (OBPP) is a school-based program designed to prevent or reduce school bullying by identifying and focusing on three aspects of a school: schoolwide, classroom, and the individual. At the *school level*, the first step of the program is to identify bullies and bullying victims [53–55]. School faculty and staff administer the OBPP questionnaire to students to assess the prevalence and characteristics of bullying occurring among the student body [53–55]. Then, the school staff establishes a committee to implement training for all faculty and staff members to address bullying. Finally, faculty and staff develop curricula for all students that highlight the schoolwide rules against bullying, while promoting the importance of mutual respect and healthy relations among students. Within the *classroom*, teachers deliver several anti-bullying lessons or oversee student meetings about school bullying and peer relations [53–55]. Teachers also extend communication and discussions about school bullying with parents. At the *individual level*, students may be individually identified as a bully or bullying victim to having regularly scheduled meetings to discuss and address why the bullying is occurring and what can be done to resolve the violence. Via these mechanisms, the OBPP attempts to reorganize the school to decrease the occurrence of bullying.

Although the OBPP is generally viewed by school administrators as successful, there have been limited studies that examine the effectiveness and the limitations of anti-bullying programs, and inconsistent findings in these studies are common [see e.g., 56–58]. Because the definition of bullying is complex and relative [53, 59, 60], the OBPP may not address all forms of perceived bullying. In this context, the perception of violence, injury, and victimization is primarily based on adult definitions and understandings of bullying, which may lead to under- or over-monitoring of violent student behavior [59–62]. In other words, a school administrator, faculty, and staff interpretations may influence the utilization of bullying prevention policies. Intimidation based on race, ethnicity, gender, religion, socioeconomic status, social class, physical ability, and sexual orientation are sometimes excluded from definitions of bullying and are therefore not addressed by anti-bullying policies [53, 59, 60]. Of course, this may be complicated by the relative and subjective definitions of each student, teacher, administrator, and parent's view of bullying.

There are three recommendations associated with social inequality that should be considered by schools that incorporate OBPP practices. First, for OBPP to be successful, administrators and teachers must be trained to understand and identify behavioral problems and detrimental treatment in their classrooms; however, vulnerable and marginalized students are more likely to attend disadvantaged schools that are less likely to have well-qualified teachers who could properly address the problems of bullying [59, 60]. Second, as noted throughout this book, vulnerable and marginalized students are more likely to attend schools with increased levels of disorder, violence, and crime. Therefore, community disorder, violence, and crime may impose serious limitations on the effectiveness of OBPP practices because bullying is often constructed as "minor" and not pressing in such schools [59, 60]. Third, cultural disparities could pose a hurdle for OBPP practices. As discussed, inconsistent definitions of school bullying, as well as the complexities associated with misinterpreted interpersonal behaviors, are embedded with social and cultural understandings [59, 60]. Thus, OBPP facilitators should consider and knowledgeable of the social and cultural distinctions associated with defining and responding to school bullying.

Implications for Restorative Justice in Schools

Originally applied to the criminal justice system, *restorative justice* interventions have attempted to repair the harm caused by criminal offenses while preventing further violence and crime; this is generally accomplished through mediation and conferences that reconcile the conflict between offenders, victims, and other community members [63–66]. The importance of communication between offenders, victims, and the community affected by the violence is perceived as a resolution that facilitates closure for the victim and responsibility taken by the offender [63–66]. Allowing the offender to emphasize, discuss, and take responsibility for the violence or harmful act is an important aspect of the restorative justice process as well as minimize the reoccurrence of such behavior [63–66]. Communication between the victim and offender allows the offender to see how violence harms others and as well as enable the victim, offender, and community stakeholders impacted by the violent act to make a collaborative decision toward addressing the injury [63–66]. Restorative justice practices are gaining attention and utilization within schools as an alternative for stringent school punishment practices [63, 65, 66].

Instead of excluding and punishing, restorative justice in schools sees violence as a form of conflict and acts proactively to find alternative ways to handle conflicts, such as peer mediation, or other forms of settlement-directed talking, such as restorative conferencing and peacemaking circles [63, 67, 68]. Completely contrary to the disciplinary practice of student exclusion, restorative approaches in schools focus on relationships, shifting from punishment and isolation to reconciliation and community [63, 67, 68]. Some argue that restorative justice is best applied to the school context because of the nature of relationships where students see each other day after day, where encounters can turn dangerous if not adequately managed [63, 67, 68]. Within a restorative justice perspective, misbehavior is viewed as a violation of the relationship between teachers, administrators, and/or other students [63, 67, 68]. To restore the harm of such a violation, the offending student and the individual whose trust was violated must reconcile and relationship mended. The importance of building and maintaining positive relationships, especially between members of a school community, is continually stressed [63, 67, 68]. Primary restorative practices involve the entire school community and aim at establishing a values ethic, as well as skill base, for developing relational ecologies and resolving differences in respectful and caring ways. Secondary restorative practices address specific behaviors that disrupt the harmony and social relations of classrooms (e.g., problem-solving circles), hallways (e.g., corridor conferences) and playgrounds (e.g., peer mediations). Tertiary restorative practices are the most intensive, often responding to serious harm, and involve all those affected (including families, professionals, fellow students, and others affected) in a face-to-face restorative justice process [67].

There are three recommendations associated with social inequality that should be considered by schools that utilize restorative justice practices. First, because restorative justice often includes community stakeholders, such as parents, siblings, and the like, school administrators should be mindful of the community attitudes and beliefs about socioeconomic and social status, family cohesion and interactions, sex, sexual orientation, gender identity, gender expression, race, ethnicity, immigration status, religion, disabilities, and special health needs. As noted throughout this book, it is plausible that xenophobia, homophobia, sexism, racism, classism, and the like could be reflective of the community environment and parental beliefs that may be transmitted through youth aggression. Second, because communication and empathy are essential toward successful restorative justice practices between all parties involved, socioeconomic, social, and cultural barriers and misunderstandings may impede the restorative justice process between participants. Third, as presented throughout this book, school administrators and teachers should be mindful of the potential tensions and conflict between affluent and poor students, heteronormative and LGBTQ students, White and racial/ethnic minority students, native and foreign-born students, etcetera, because these social and cultural inequalities and disparities could result in harassment, victimization, and aggression. School administrators and faculty should learn the nuances and complexities associated with the challenges and tensions that marginalized and vulnerable youth face at school.

Considering Educational Success, Progress, and Well-being with Safety

Any pursuits of ameliorating violence and ensuring the safety of marginalized and vulnerable youth within a school, it is essential to also ensure the educational success and progress of this disadvantaged student population. Historical and contemporary research examines the ongoing debate about stratification and inequality and their influence on U.S. public education [41–43, 45]. Although these studies describe the role of schools in preserving and reproducing cultural, social, and economic inequalities, they have not sufficiently accounted for the role of school safety in perpetuating and/or disrupting such inequities. Schools are potentially a stage in the process of incorporation and stratification. Marginalized and vulnerable students' experiences with school safety help to facilitate this process, increasing the odds of maintaining the already existing status quo. If schools are charged with being safe havens that nurture the potential for all youth to shape their world, then understanding marginalized and vulnerable youth experiences with school safety are imperative. In this section, we highlighted how school safety approaches (i.e., zero-tolerance and control, schoolwide positive behavioral interventions and support, communal schools, Olweus bullying prevention, and restorative justice) could benefit from including factors associated with social inequality to pursue marginalized and vulnerable students' safety and well-being while at school.

Although we discussed important factors associated with social inequality for distinct school safety approaches or programs, three fundamental factors matter across school safety programs, and that warrant highlighting, listed below. First, the hurdles and barriers that marginalized and vulnerable youth face at school in terms of their safety and learning intersect with the inequities linked to religion, gender, sexual orientation, race and ethnicity, immigration, and socioeconomic and social status. The identities that the children of immigrants encapsulate are dynamic and complex. School safety program leaders often should be mindful not to stereotype or homogenize the children of immigrants but consider the myriad of disadvantages that marginalized and vulnerable students endure at school. Second, the social, cultural, and political debate about if and how to address social inequality is often heated and controversial. Unfortunately, the unintended consequences may make the marginalized and vulnerable students susceptible to additional harassment and victimization from faculty and administrators who are responsible for all students' safety. School safety program leaders should be mindful of such social and cultural biases. Third, because schools are a site of education and socialization for marginalized and vulnerable students, the effect of school violence and victimization as well as punishment and discipline could have disproportional negative effects for this disadvantaged youth population.

Highlighting Conclusions

This book sought to highlight how inequality is important to consider understanding, researching, and addressing school bullying and ensuring safe learning environments for all youth. The research presented in this book reveals that there are important advances to the field that can be achieved by attempting to better understand the correlates, contexts, and consequences of social inequality in the relationship between school bullying, victimization, violence, safety, and educational progress and success. We will summarize the highlight of each of the chapters of this book.

In Chap. 2, "The Relevance of the Social-Ecological Model and the Significance of Inequality," we detailed how inequality matters when utilizing the social-ecological framework. We highlighted the significance of social stratification and inequality when investigating the connections between social environment and youth development. We laid the conceptual groundwork for us to consider how (1) social position (e.g., race, class, and gender), (2) social stratification (e.g., biased treatment), (3) promoting or inhibiting environments (e.g., school), (4) adaptive culture and current demands (e.g., assimilation or acculturation), (5) youth characteristics (e.g., age, psychological characteristics), and (6) family (e.g., structure, functioning) are important when understanding the role inequality has in school bullying.

In Chapt. 3, "Status Matters: How Socioeconomic and Social Statuses are Associated with Bullying," we demonstrated how inequalities in socioeconomic and social statuses are associated with bullying victimization. A student's popularity and friendships or social networks can be linked to the likelihood of the student experiencing bullying victimization and aggression at school. Additionally, characteristics correlated to student social status also influence the likelihood of school bullying victimization.

In Chap. 4, "The Role of the Family: Parents/Guardians, Siblings, Cohesion and Interactions," we depicted how the inequality associated with the role of the family, specifically parents/guardians, siblings, cohesion, and interactions are linked with the likelihood of being bullied. For example, on the one hand, bullied youth who have strong and intimate bonds or relationships with their parents/guardians might have more favorable adjustment outcomes than would otherwise be the case. On the other hand, family factors, such as negative adult and sibling influences, lack of parental involvement, bullying among siblings, and lack of parental support, maltreatment, and unhealthy family interactions are associated with bullying victimization.

In Chap. 5, "Sex, Sexual Orientation, Gender Identity, and Gender Expression: Definitions and Implications for Marginalization," we demonstrated that the inequalities associated with sex, sexual orientation, gender identity, and gender expression contribute to being bullied at school. For instance, LGBTQ students experience increased levels of physical harassment, verbal intimidation, and social isolation, as well as biased treatment from faculty, administrators, and staff.

In Chap. 6, "The Color of School Bullying Victimization: Race, Ethnicity, Immigration, and Religion," we explained how racial, ethnic, immigration, and religious inequality are associated with school bullying. We also highlighted the ways that social, cultural, and political climate or school contexts also impact students' experiences with bullying. For example, since the events of September 11, 2001, Muslim and Arab American youth have reported a dramatic increase in bullying victimization, harassment, and verbal and physical threats while in school.

In Chap. 7, "Bullying and Youth with Disabilities and Special Health Need: Victimizing Students with Physical, Emotional, and Learning Disorders," we discussed how inequality linked to disabilities and special health needs contributes to an increased likelihood of being bullied in school. For example, bullying incidents involving youth with disabilities are difficult to identify because these youth are less likely to have learned about abuse awareness and potential responses, which makes detection and reporting of bullying among this population a serious concern.

In Chap. 8, "Bullying and Victimization of Youth in the Court System," we discussed the experiences of bullying and peer victimization of youth who are involved in the juvenile justice system and youth who are involved in the child welfare system. We highlighted how societal, community, institutional, group, and individual contexts might impact the bullying experiences of these adolescents.

At the Current Historical Moment

As we are completing this book for submission, we would like to acknowledge the current historical moment by discussing three significant socio-cultural events directly connected to our book about school bullying and inequality: COVID-19; Black Lives Matter movement; and, the 2020 Supreme Court Ruling on DACA. This section will provide a brief discussion about how this current historical moment could mark a turning point that highlights the need to address the vulnerabilities that the children daily endure in communities and schools in regards to bullying.

There are three overarching factors in thinking about how COVID-19 is relevant to this topic of school bullying and inequality: the US justice system, education, and hate crime. Miller and colleagues' [69] provide a broad overview of how COVID-19 is influencing the relationship between immigration and the US justice system. In essence, they argue that the vulnerabilities and inequalities immigrants and their children faced prior to COVID-19 are only being exacerbated. Concerns have been raised about aggressive policy changes, enforcement actions, immigrant detention, and deportation practices in response to and during the COVID-19 outbreak [69]. All of these actions are having detrimental consequences on immigrants and their children in regards to their safety, health, and overall well-being. Second, Viner and colleagues' [70] offer a broad overview how COVID-19 is influencing educational systems in the US and globally. They describe how schools have basically been shut down. At this moment, it remains unknown when and how public schools will even reopen. It is easy to predict that how we understand "school safety" in regards to violence and crime will now include conceptualizations of public health and well-being for the entire school community in a post COVID-19 era. Third, Tessler and colleagues' [71] offer a broad overview how COVID-19 is exacerbating Asian American vulnerabilities associated with hate crimes and negative biases. It is evident that COVID-19 has elevated the risks of Asian Americans to hate crimes and business vandalism to their businesses. Asian Americans have historically been viewed as perpetually foreign no matter how long they have lived in the US. It is therefore argued that present-day socio-cultural beliefs constructing Asian Americans as foreign and diseased are historical and persistent [71]. The hate crimes and negative biases against Asian Americans in the time of COVID-19 highlight how additional burdens of anxiety, economic instability, and the risk of violence and victimization are imposed upon Asian Americans. Of course, understandings of school safety and how we pursue such understandings in a post-COVID-19 context remain unknown, especially in regards to the implications for the children of immigrants.

The social and cultural protests around the recent tragic deaths of George Floyd, Breonna Taylor, and Ahmaud Arbery and the calls for racial justice have been magnified through civil unrest throughout the US and world. Such protests have centered around the "Black Lives Matter" movement. Taylor [72] offer a broad overview of the "Black Lives Matter" movement; however, the civil unrest and protest within the US has re-centered historical and systemic social problems about racial/ethnic inequality and oppression within justice systems, including the growing presence of law enforcement in schools. As noted in this book, discriminatory treatment and inequitable access to educational resources for racial/ethnic minority students are historical and persistent with detrimental consequences. Social, public, and media discourses about defunding law enforcement and terminating the utilization of school resource officers across US schools have emerged from the protests about racial/ethnic inequity. Without a doubt if law enforcement is defunded and police and school resource officer presence within schools are ended, this would have profound, fundamental, and unclear implications for school safety overall, especially for racial/ethnic minorities.

In June 2020, the Supreme Court blocked the Trump administration's attempt to end DACA, citing efforts to end the program as "arbitrary and capricious." DACA beneficiaries breathed a sigh a relief as the Supreme Court decision allowed them to continue to stay in school, work, and remain with relatives while being protected from deportation. However, the Supreme Court decision also paved the way for the Trump administration to try and end DACA once again as long as they follow the appropriate process. It remains unknown if the administration will pursue ending the program during an election year, particularly given bi-partisan support for DACA. Within schools, the court's decision leaves undocumented students, as well as the children of immigrants, with uncertain futures. As noted, attempts to repeal DACA combined with heightened immigration enforcement have had chilling effects on students, families, and schools. As the US edges closer to the next presidential election, it will important to explore the implications of DACA and its potential repeal for the children of immigrants.

We have noted throughout this book that social, cultural, and political contexts frame how we understand the associations between education, safety, and school bullying and inequality in the US. It is uncertain if and how COVID-19, the "Black Lives Matter" movement, and the 2020 Supreme Court Ruling on DACA will influence the evident vulnerabilities that the children of immigrants daily endure in communities and schools. Nevertheless, we have a duty and responsibility to highlight these historic events in regards to immigration and school safety.

Conclusion

We encourage future research to further expand our understanding of social inequality, bullying, victimization, violence, safety, and justice for marginalized and vulnerable youth. The increasing diversity of students provides both a challenge and an opportunity for the U.S. educational system. As marginalized and vulnerable youth graduate high school and college, enter the labor force, become voters, form families, and ultimately lead the United States into its future, research on such future work promises to provide important opportunities for theoretical advancement on democracy, education, and justice.

References

1. Espelage, D. L. (2016). Sexual orientation and gender identity in schools: A call for more research in school psychology—No more excuses. *Journal of School Psychology, 54*, 5–8.
2. Birkett, M., Espelage, D. L., & Koenig, B. (2009). LGB and questioning students in schools: The moderating effects of homophobic bullying and school climate on negative outcomes. *Journal of Youth and Adolescence, 38*(7), 989–1000.

3. Kahle, L. (2017). Are sexual minorities more at risk? Bullying victimization among lesbian, gay, bisexual, and questioning youth. *Journal of Interpersonal Violence*, 0886260517718830.
4. Kahle, L. (2018). Feminist and queer criminology: A vital place for theorizing LGBTQ youth. *Sociology Compass, 12*(3), e12564.
5. Pascoe, C. J. (2011). *Dude, you're a fag: Masculinity and sexuality in high school*. University of California Press.
6. Meyer, E. (2008). A feminist reframing of bullying and harassment: Transforming schools through critical pedagogy. *McGill Journal of Education/Revue des sciences de l'éducation de McGill, 43*(1), 33–48.
7. Peguero, A. A., & Bondy, J. M. (2020). The importance of immigration with future research about school safety. *Race and Justice, 10*(3), 247–268.
8. Schwartz, A. E., Stiefel, L., & Rothbart, M. W. (2016). Do top dogs rule in middle school? Evidence on bullying, safety, and belonging. *American Educational Research Journal, 53*(5), 1450–1484.
9. Zembylas, M. (2010). Teachers' emotional experiences of growing diversity and multiculturalism in schools and the prospects of an ethic of discomfort. *Teachers and Teaching: Theory and Practice, 16*(6), 703–716.
10. Zembylas, M. (2012). Transnationalism, migration and emotions: Implications for education. *Globalisation, Societies and Education, 10*(2), 163–179.
11. Espelage, D. L. (2014). Ecological theory: Preventing youth bullying, aggression, and victimization. *Theory Into Practice, 53*(4), 257–264.
12. Gonzales, R. G. (2015). *Lives in limbo: Undocumented and coming of age in America*. Berkeley, CA: University of California Press.
13. Foucault, M. (1977). Discipline and punish: The birth of the prison. Vintage.
14. Simon, J. (2007). *Governing through crime: How the war on crime transformed American democracy and created a culture of fear*. Oxford University Press.
15. Crenshaw, K., Ocen, P., & Nanda, J. (2015). *Black girls matter: Pushed out, overpoliced, and underprotected*. New York, NY: Center for Intersectionality and Social Policy Studies, Columbia University.
16. Morris, M. (2016). *Pushout: The criminalization of black girls in schools*. New York: The New Press.
17. Portillos, E. L., González, J. C., & Peguero, A. A. (2012). Crime control strategies in school: Chicanas'/os' perceptions and criminalization. *The Urban Review, 44*(2), 171–188.
18. Rios, V. M. (2011). *Punished: Policing the lives of black and Latino boys*. NYU Press.
19. Rios, V. M. (2017). *Human targets: Schools, police, and the criminalization of Latino youth*. University of Chicago Press.
20. Noguera, P. A. (2009). *The trouble with black boys:... And other reflections on race, equity, and the future of public education*. San Francisco, CA: Jossey-Bass.
21. Peguero, A. A., & Shekarkhar, Z. (2011). Latino/a student misbehavior and school punishment. *Hispanic Journal of Behavioral Sciences, 33*(1), 54–70.
22. Muschert, G. W., & Peguero, A. A. (2010). The Columbine effect and school anti-violence policy. *Research in Social Problems and Public Policy, 17*, 117–148.
23. Kupchik, A. (2010). *Homeroom security: School discipline in an age of fear*. New York: NYU Press.
24. Addington, L. A. (2009). Cops and cameras: Public school security as a policy response to Columbine. *American Behavioral Scientist, 52*(10), 1426–1446.
25. Muschert, G. W., Henry, S., Bracy, N. L., & Peguero, A. A. (2013). *Responding to school violence: Confronting the Columbine effect*. Boulder, CO: Lynne Rienner Publishers.
26. Bradshaw, C. P. (2013). Preventing bullying through positive behavioral interventions and supports (PBIS): A multitiered approach to prevention and integration. *Theory Into Practice, 52*(4), 288–295.

27. Bradshaw, C. P., Koth, C. W., Bevans, K. B., Ialongo, N., & Leaf, P. J. (2008). The impact of school-wide positive behavioral interventions and supports (PBIS) on the organizational health of elementary schools. *School Psychology Quarterly, 23*(4), 462.
28. Bradshaw, C. P., Koth, C. W., Thornton, L. A., & Leaf, P. J. (2009). Altering school climate through school-wide positive behavioral interventions and supports: Findings from a group-randomized effectiveness trial. *Prevention Science, 10*(2), 100.
29. Simonsen, B., Sugai, G., & Negron, M. (2008). Schoolwide positive behavior supports: Primary systems and practices. *Teaching Exceptional Children, 40*(6), 32–40.
30. Sprague, J. R., & Golly, A. (2005). *Best behavior: Building positive behavior support in schools*. Longmont, CO: Sopris-West.
31. Sugai, G., & Horner, R. (2010). School-wide positive behavior support: Establishing a continuum of evidence based practices. *Journal of Evidence-Based Practices for Schools, 11*(1), 62–83.
32. Peguero, A. A., & Bondy, J. M. (2015). Schools, justice, and immigrant students: Segmented assimilation, race, ethnicity, gender, and perceptions of fairness and order. *Teachers College Record, 117*(7), n7.
33. Peguero, A. A., Bondy, J. M., & Shekarkhar, Z. (2017). Punishing Latina/o youth: School justice, fairness, order, dropping out, and gender disparities. *Hispanic Journal of Behavioral Sciences, 39*(1), 98–125.
34. Shedd, C. (2015). *Unequal city: Race, schools, and perceptions of injustice*. Russell Sage Foundation.
35. Gottfredson, D. C. (2001). *Schools and delinquency*. New York: Cambridge University Press.
36. Gottfredson, D. C. (2017). Prevention research in schools: Past, present, and future. *Criminology & Public Policy, 16*(1), 7–27.
37. Gottfredson, G. D., Gottfredson, D. C., Payne, A. A., & Gottfredson, N. C. (2005). School climate predictors of school disorder: Results from a national study of delinquency prevention in schools. *Journal of Research in Crime and Delinquency, 42*(4), 412–444.
38. Payne, A. A. (2004). *School community and disorder: Communal schools, student bonding, delinquency, and victimization*. El Paso, TX: LFB Scholarly Publishing.
39. Payne, A. A. (2008). A multilevel analysis of the relationships among communal school organization, student bonding, and delinquency. *Journal of Research in Crime and Delinquency, 45*(4), 429–455.
40. Payne, A. A., Gottfredson, D. C., & Gottfredson, G. D. (2003). Schools as communities: The relationships among communal school organization, student bonding, and school disorder. *Criminology, 41*(3), 749–778.
41. Kozol, J. (2005). *The shame of the nation: The restoration of apartheid schooling in America*. Broadway Books.
42. Kozol, J. (2012). *Savage inequalities: Children in America's schools*. Broadway Books.
43. Lareau, A. (2011). *Unequal childhoods: Class, race, and family life*. Univ of California Press.
44. Lewis, A. E. (2003). *Race in the schoolyard: Reproducing the color line in school 2003b New Brunswick*. New Brunzwick, NJ: Rutgers University Press.
45. Lewis, A. E., & Diamond, J. B. (2017). *Despite the best intentions: How racial inequality thrives in good schools*. Oxford University Press.
46. Kao, G., Vaquera, E., & Goyette, K. (2013). *Education and immigration*. John Wiley & Sons.
47. Lee, S. J. (2009). *Unraveling the" model minority" stereotype: Listening to Asian American youth*. New York: Teachers College Press.
48. Lee, J., & Zhou, M. (2015). *The Asian American achievement paradox*. New York: Russell Sage Foundation.
49. Peguero, A. A. (2008). Is immigrant status relevant in school violence research? An analysis with Latino students. *Journal of School Health, 78*(7), 397–404.
50. Peguero, A. A. (2009). Victimizing the children of immigrants: Latino and Asian American student victimization. *Youth & Society, 41*(2), 186–208.

51. Peguero, A. A. (2013). An adolescent victimization immigrant paradox? School-based routines, lifestyles, and victimization across immigration generations. *Journal of Youth and Adolescence, 42*(11), 1759–1773.
52. Peguero, A. A. (2008). Bullying victimization and extracurricular activity. *Journal of School Violence, 7*(3), 71–85.
53. Espelage, D. L., & Swearer, S. M. (2010). *Bullying in North American schools*. Routledge.
54. Olweus, D. (1993). *Bullying at school: What we know and what we can do*. Oxford, UK: Blackwell Publishers.
55. Olweus, D., Limber, S., & Mihalic, S. (1999). *Bullying prevention program: Blueprints for violence prevention, book nine*. Boulder, CO: Center for the Study and Prevention of Violence.
56. Farrington, D. P., & Ttofi, M. M. (2009). School-based programs to reduce bullying and victimization. *Campbell systematic reviews, 5*(1), i–148.
57. Ttofi, M. M., & Farrington, D. P. (2011). Effectiveness of school-based programs to reduce bullying: A systematic and meta-analytic review. *Journal of Experimental Criminology, 7*(1), 27–56.
58. Mishna, F. (2008). An overview of the evidence on bullying prevention and intervention programs. *Brief Treatment and Crisis Intervention, 8*(4), 327.
59. Hong, J. S. (2009). Feasibility of the Olweus bullying prevention program in low-income schools. *Journal of School Violence, 8*(1), 81–97.
60. Peguero, A. A. (2012). Schools, bullying, and inequality: Intersecting factors and complexities with the stratification of youth victimization at school. *Sociology Compass, 6*(5), 402–412.
61. Safran, E. R. (2007). Bullying behavior, bully prevention programs, and gender. *Journal of Emotional Abuse, 7*(4), 43–67.
62. Vaillancourt, T., McDougall, P., Hymel, S., Krygsman, A., Miller, J., Stiver, K., & Davis, C. (2008). Bullying: Are researchers and children/youth talking about the same thing? *International Journal of Behavioral Development, 32*(6), 486–495.
63. Gonzalez, T. (2012). Keeping kids in schools: Restorative justice, punitive discipline, and the school to prison pipeline. *JL & Educ., 41*, 281.
64. Lockhart, A., Zammit, L., Charboneau, R., Owens, R., & Ross, R. (2005). *Restorative justice: Transforming society*. Inclusion Press.
65. Stinchcomb, J. B., Bazemore, G., & Riestenberg, N. (2006). Beyond zero tolerance: Restoring justice in secondary schools. *Youth Violence and Juvenile Justice, 4*(2), 123–147.
66. Pavelka, S. (2013). Practices and policies for implementing restorative justice within schools. *The Prevention Researcher, 20*(1), 15–18.
67. Morrison, B. E., & Vaandering, D. (2012). Restorative justice: Pedagogy, praxis, and discipline. *Journal of School Violence, 11*(2), 138–155.
68. Payne, A. A., & Welch, K. (2013). Restorative justice in schools: The influence of race on restorative discipline. *Youth & Society, 47*(4), 539–564.
69. Miller, H. V., Ripepi, M., Ernstes, A. M., & Peguero, A. A. (2020). Immigration policy and justice in the era of COVID-19. *American Journal of Criminal Justice*, 1–17.
70. Viner, R. M., Russell, S. J., Croker, H., Packer, J., Ward, J., Stansfield, C., Booy, R. et al. (2020). School closure and management practices during coronavirus outbreaks including COVID-19: A rapid systematic review. *The Lancet Child & Adolescent Health 4*.
71. Tessler, H., Choi, M., & Kao, G. (2020). The anxiety of being Asian American: Hate crimes and negative biases during the COVID-19 pandemic. *American Journal of Criminal Justice*, 1–11.
72. Taylor, K.-Y. (2016). *From #BlackLivesMatter to black liberation*. Haymarket Books.

Index

A
Administrators, 114–116
Adolescent bullying, 44, 45
Adverse outcomes, 91
Aggression, 91
Aggressive sex, 55, 106
Americans with Disabilities Act of 1990, 89
Attention-deficit/hyperactivity disorder, 85
Autism spectrum disorder (ASD), 86, 87

B
Backlash effects, 77
Biological sex, 55, 62
Black Lives Matter, 126
Bullying and aggressive behaviors, 104
Bullying victimization, 55
Bystanders, 26, 27

C
Centers for Disease Control and Prevention, 1, 85
Cerebral palsy, 86
Child Trends, 100
Child Welfare League of America, 101
Child welfare system, 100, 101
Children's Society, 15
Code of the Street, 75
Collective efficacy, 46
Communal schools, 119, 120
Community, 28, 29, 46, 59, 74, 75, 90, 103
Complexities, 48, 62, 63, 93, 94, 106, 107
Conduct disorder, 87
Conventional school violence research, 3
Court system
  bullying, 99
  child welfare system, 100, 101
  complexities, 106, 107
  delinquency, 100
  juvenile justice system, 100
  peer victimization, 99
COVID-19, 126
Culture, 45

D
Delinquency, 100
Disability harassment, 89
Disciplinary society, 116
Dominance, 91

E
Educational faculty, 114–116
Educational success, 123, 124
Emotional/behavioral disorders, 86, 87
Empathy, 61
Ethnicity, 70, 71
Exposure, 33

F
Family cohesion, 44, 45
Family conflict, 44, 45
Family functioning, 44
Family-level factors, 48
Family systems framework, 44
Federal laws, 89

A. A. Peguero, J. S. Hong, *School Bullying*, Springer Series on Child and Family Studies, https://doi.org/10.1007/978-3-030-64367-6

G
Gay, Lesbian and Straight Education Network (GLSEN), 56
Gender, 14
Gender expression, 56, 57
Gender identity, 56, 57
Gender non-conforming, 63
Guardianship, 33

H
Hearing loss, 86
Homophobic bullying, 55, 57, 62, 63

I
Immigrant paradox, 80
Immigration, 69, 71, 72, 126
Institutional level, 59, 60, 75, 76
  factors, 93
  level, 29, 30
Intellectual disability, 86
Intersectionality, 4
Islamophobia, 72

J
Juvenile justice system, 100

L
Law enforcement, 126
Learning Disabilities Association of America, 88
Learning disability, 86, 88
Learning disorders, 86, 88
Learning environments, 124
Lesbian, gay, and bisexual, transgender, and sexually questioning (LGBTQ), 5, 8, 56

M
Macro-political context, 115
Macrosystem level factors, 18
Micro lived experiences, 115
Multi-disciplinary approach, 5

N
National Gay and Lesbian Task Force and National Center for Transgender Equality, 63
National School Climate Survey, 57

O
Olweus Bullying Prevention Program (OBPP), 120, 121
Opportunity theory, 32

P
Parental support, 42
Parents/guardians, 41, 42
Parent–teacher collaborations, 42
Parent-youth relations, 41
Peer victimization, 91, 99
Physical disabilities
  adolescents, 86
  bully victimization, 86
  bullying, 86
  child abuse, 85
  children, 86
  chronic conditions, 86
  complexities, 93, 94
  corporal injury, 85
  definition, 86
  developmental delays, 86
  emotional/behavioral disorders, 87
  impairments, 86
  learning disorders, 88
  peer victimization, 86
  prevalence of childhood, 86
  social-ecological context, 86
  types, 86
Policymakers, 114–116
Progress, 123, 124
Proximity, 33
Psychosocial characteristics, 92

R
Race, 70, 71
Rehabilitation Act of 1973, 89
Relational aggression, 56, 62
Religion, 72
Restorative justice interventions, 122, 123
Role of family
  adolescence, 39
  adolescent bullying, 44, 45
  aggression, 40
  American family structure, 39
  complexities, 48
  cyberbullying, 40
  definition, 39
  environmental context, 40
  family cohesion, 44, 45
  family conflict, 44, 45
  guardians, 41, 42

parents, 41, 42
role of sibling, 40
sibling bullying, 40
siblings, 42–44
social-ecological framework, 40
social-ecological perspective, 39

S
Safe School Climate Act, 91
Scholars, 62
School bullying, 62
biological sex, 8
broader social environmental factors, 2
contexts of socialization, 1
disabilities, 9
disparities, 2
diverse social factors, 2
factors, 1–2
family factors, 8
gender identity, 8
growing significance, 5, 6
immigrant youth, 9
inequality, 2–6
low-income youth, 7
patterns, 9
peer victimization, 10
psychosocial outcomes, 7
psychosocial problems, 9
racial and ethnic minority, 9
research literature, 10
sexual minority, 2
sexual/physical violence, 8
social-ecological approach, 2, 10
social-ecological framework, 6, 8
social environments, 6
social networks, 7
social skills, 8
social stratification, 6
socioeconomic and social status, 2, 7, 10
special health needs, 9
stressful experience, 7
students' experiences, 2
transgender status, 8
victimization, 2, 9, 10
violence, 10
youth development, 6
youth violence, 1, 2
School bullying victimization
complexities, 79, 80
differential patterns, 69
ethnicity, 70, 71
immigrant youth, 69
immigration, 71, 72
racial and ethnic disparities, 69–71
religion, 72
social-ecological framework, 70
School climate, 16
School environment, 16
School level, 120
Schoolwide Positive Behavior Interventions and Supports (SWPBIS), 118, 119
Secure Our Schools Act of 2000, 116
Sex differences, 55, 56
Sexual bullying, 59
Sexual orientation, 55–57, 62
Siblings, 42–44
Social cognition, 46
Social control, 116, 117
Social-ecological framework
adaptive culture and demands, 16, 17
adolescent bullying, 45
bullying victimization, 27
community, 28, 29, 46, 59, 74, 75, 90
complexities, 18, 19
family, 18, 45
group-level, 31, 32
groups, 46, 47, 60, 61, 77, 78, 104, 105
individual level, 32, 33, 47, 61, 62, 78, 79, 92, 105, 106
institutional level, 29, 30, 59, 60, 91, 104
multiple level factors, 14
peer group, 91, 92
power imbalance, 13
promoting/inhibiting environments, 15, 16
school bullying, 13
social environment, 14
social inequality, 13
societal level, 27, 28, 45, 58, 73, 74, 89, 90, 102
social position, 14
social stratification, 13, 15
youth characteristics, 17
Social environment, 62, 103, 124
Social inequality, 113, 114, 124
Social learning theory, 103
Social networks, 26, 27
Social organization, 46
Social position, 14
Social stratification, 13, 15, 18
Social support, 92
Socio-cultural events, 125
Socioeconomic and social statuses, 124
affluence, 24
aggressive/dominant behavior, 25
behavioral norms, 25
bystanders, 26, 27
complexities, 33, 34

Socioeconomic and social statuses (*cont.*)
expectations, 25
friendships, 26, 27
implications, 24
individual measures, 24
likelihood of victimization, 23
low-income families, 24
poverty, 24
prestige-based indicator, 24
resource-based indicator, 24
role of power, 24
school bullying, 23, 24
school-level, 24
social-ecological framework, 24, 25
social hierarchy, 25
social networks, 23, 26, 27
social sanctions, 25
youth violence, 24
Socio-political context, 115
Staff, 114–116
Student Civil Rights Act of 2007 (SB777), 58
Suitable target, 32
Supreme Court decision, 127

T
Transgender, 63

U
United Nations Children's Fund, 85
U.S. Department of Health and Human Services, 100
US justice system, 126

V
Victimization, 62
Violence, 63
Vision impairment, 86
Visual impairment, 93

W
Well-being, 123, 124

Y
Youth development, 124
Youth violence, 1

Z
Zero-tolerance, 116, 117

The manufacturer's authorised representative in the EU is Springer
Nature Customer Service Centre GmbH, Europaplatz 3, 69115 Heidelberg,
Germany. If you have any concerns regarding our products, please
contact ProductSafety@springernature.com

Printed and bound by CPI Group (UK) Ltd, Croydon, CR0 4YY
30/09/2026
02225470-0010